A History of Physical

(The Story of the British Association of Rheumatology and Rehabilitation)

Geoffrey O Storey

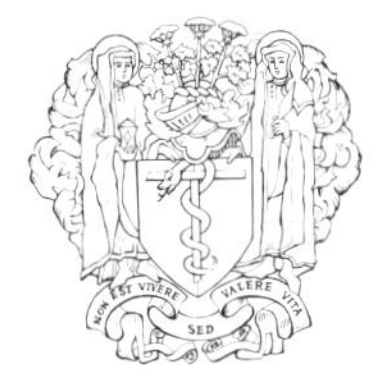

Royal Society of Medicine Services Limited

Royal Society of Medicine Services Limited
1 Wimpole Street London W1M 8AE
8 East 60th Street New York NY 10022

British Library Cataloguing in Publication Data
Storey, Geoffrey
A history of physical medicine.
I. Title
616.723

ISBN 1853151688
ISBN 185315167X pbk

Editorial and production services by Diane Crofter-Harris, Devizes, Wiltshire

Phototypeset by Dobbie Typesetting Limited, Tavistock, Devon

Printed in Great Britain by Henry Ling Ltd at the Dorset Press, Dorchester, Dorset

Contents

List of Illustrations

To my wife

Preface

Rheumatology in Great Britain and Ireland has undergone many changes in the last 50 years. The name of the specialty has varied and has included Physical Medicine and subsequently Rheumatology and Rehabilitation. It has only recently separated from Rehabilitation, though there remain close links between the two disciplines, and their separation is an amiable divorce. There has been a similar pattern of changes in the professional and scientific societies and also in the journals for the specialty. There is now one society, The British Society for Rheumatology, with its accompanying journal, *The British Journal of Rheumatology*. But it seems only yesterday that there were two societies; the Heberden Society and the British Association for Rheumatology and Rehabilitation. The origins and course of the Heberden Society has been previously described by Dr John Moll. The history of the British Association for Rheumatology and Rehabilitation, affectionately known by its acronym of BARR, together with its earlier entities is outlined in this book by Dr Geoffrey Storey.

Hospital medicine in the City and East London has been in flux for many years with constant changes in the hospitals and their affiliations to each other. Dr Storey was my immediate predecessor in Hackney, and he worked at a number of the medical institutions in East London; these included Hackney Hospital, Bethnal Green Hospital, and the London Hospital. Only the London Hospital will continue into the future. His experience of the changes in the organisation of clinical practice reflects the reorganisation and changes in the specialist societies which he elegantly chronicles in this monograph.

Change is an inevitable part of life, including our professional careers, and is invariably a force working for the good of patients and physicians. Of course we rarely feel the advantages of changes in the organisation of clinical practice when they are taking place, and tend to focus on the problems of new arrangements. Dr Storey's account of rheumatological personalities and politics throughout the existence of BARR places the ultimate benefits of such changes into their appropriate context. He does this in an informative and relatively lighthearted manner, and gives a fascinating review of the life and times of BARR leading ultimately to the formation of a single British Society for Rheumatology.

Medical history is a subject which gathers increasing interest with passing years, and to reflect back on the events which happened early in one's career is a constant source of fascination. Geoffrey Storey does this with a deft and occasionally Delphic touch. Although it is his first book, he brings the essential authoritative style to this account of British Rheumatologists and their Society. It shows his continuing interest in clinical and academic rheumatology that has continued ever present throughout his retirement from everyday clinical practice.

Dr David L Scott
Reader in Rheumatology and Honorary Consultant Physician
St Bartholomew's Hospital Medical College
London

Introduction

On 1 January 1984, the British Association of Rheumatology and Rehabilitation (BARR) fused with the Heberden Society to form the British Society for Rheumatology (BSR). At the same time, a separate society The Medical Disability Society was formed to care for the interests of rehabilitation. The history of the Heberden Society has recently been recorded by Dr JMH Moll and it remains to trace the history of the British Association of Rheumatology and Rehabilitation. This Association started life as the British Association of Physical Medicine (BAPM) and its inaugural meeting took place on 5 May 1943. This meeting brought together doctors from several different disciplines. Although many of these interests overlap, it is possible to identify five main groups which can be discussed separately, namely: (1) The Spas; (2) Physical therapy; (3) Rheumatology; (4) Electrodiagnosis; (5) Rehabilitation. It was hoped that bringing these groups together would produce a unified specialty but perhaps these interests were always too different for this to be achieved easily at that time.

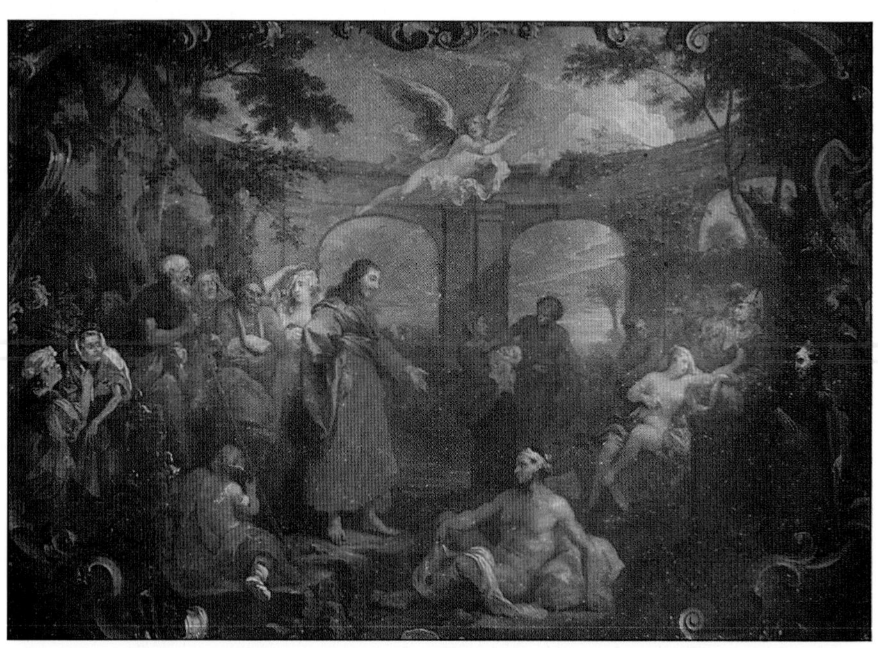

The Pool of Bethesda. William Hogarth, 1737, a mural on the Great Hall Staircase at St Bartholomew's Hospital, London. Water has always been thought to have curative properties.

Chapter 1

Origins

The Spas (Balneology, Hydrology)

Several authors have traced the history of the spas and hydrology from the earliest times, notably Sir Clifford Allbutt (1927) and MG Foster (1933). More recently GD Kersley in *The Three Rs* had given an account of the development of the spas in England particularly at Bath, and this was further expanded by Rolls in 1988 in *A Hospital for the Nation.*

In many respects, the spas may be regarded as the forerunners of 'physical medicine' and of 'rheumatology'. Bath Hospital was opened in 1742 whilst the Royal Bath Hospital in Harrogate started in 1826, Droitwich in 1836 and the Royal Devonshire Hospital Buxton began in 1858. Apart from the value of immersion in baths, it was thought at this time that the waters had specific effects when taken internally. Foster classified the various types of water and the conditions for which they might be used; the waters of Bath were particularly effective in the treatment of lead palsy. In 1905 Bain and Edgecombe analysed the waters of the spa at Harrogate for their pharmacological action.

Climatology was also felt to be important and the climate of the various spas were discussed. Bain and Edgecombe commented on the climate of Harrogate, that the winter was no worse there than the rest of the North of England but February and March were the worst months when those who could should 'elect to sojourn elsewhere'. Long stay in Harrogate would lead to an irritable condition of the nerve centres 'with subsequent lethargy and torpor'. At first, many diseases were treated at Bath, but in the early 1930s only rheumatic diseases were admitted and the hospital became the Royal National Hospital for Rheumatic Diseases with subsequent development to its present status as a centre for research and treatment of rheumatic diseases. The development at other spas followed similar lines.

The development of the spas on the continent of Europe had preceded developments in England and the first organised meeting of spa doctors in Britain seems to have been in the British Balneology and Climatological Society formed in 1895 by Dr Samual Hyde. Dr Samual Hyde (1849-1899) was born in Stalybridge (Cheshire) and he received his medical training at King's College, London, but settled in Buxton. In 1877, he became medical officer to the Peak Hydropathic and Thermal Establishment. He started the *Journal of British and Foreign Health Resorts*, as well as the British

Balneology and Climatology Society and was keen to establish physical methods of treatment as an aspect of medical science. Among his publications on medical hydrology was a paper on the *Causes and Treatment of Rheumatoid Arthritis.* He is remembered by the Samual Hyde Memorial Lecture at the Royal Society of Medicine (RSM).

The functions of the British Balneology and Climatology Society were taken over by the Section of Balneology and Climatology formed in 1909—a section of the RSM which had received its charter in 1834. A Section of Electrotherapy of the same society (formed in 1907), although mainly concerned with the development of X-rays in diagnosis, was also concerned with the development of galvanic and faradic current in diagnosis and treatment as well as the use of ultraviolet light. The Section of Balneology and Climatology, whose first president was Dr Leonard Williams, besides providing a forum for discussion of the various effects of the natural waters and the value of different climates, devoted many meetings to the diseases of the locomotor system. In March 1910 Dr Llewellyn Jones (Bath) spoke on 'Arthritis Deformans'; in 1911, CW Buckley discussed 'Osteoarthritis and its Relation to Chronic Rheumatism', and in the same year there was a discussion on 'Fibrositis'—with Llewellyn J Llewellyn in the chair (the absence of Sir William Gowers was regretted through ill health at this meeting—he had coined the term 'fibrositis' in 1904 without any real evidence for such a condition. In 1914 CW Buckley spoke on 'Painful Affections of the Shoulder'. During World War I, in 1916, there was a discussion on the treatment by physical methods of medical disabilities induced by war and in 1917 mensuration of apparatus at the Red Cross Clinic for physical treatment of officers in Great Portland Street.

During the war, as W Edgecombe reported, the spas were involved in the treatment and rehabilitation of the wounded and invalided soldiers. At Bath, treatments were given in the corporation swimming pool and patients came from several sources including the Royal Mineral Water Hospital. Rheumatic diseases were also treated as well as disabilities from war wounds, neuroses, shell-shock and neuraesthenia. Many other spas were providing similar treatments, including Buxton and Harrogate, and Strathpeffer was providing remedial exercises for various war injuries. In 1914, a survey was made on behalf of the RSM Section of Balneology and a booklet was issued to enable service medical officers to choose the right spa for the physical treatment of war injuries and the availability of hydrology, electrotherapy, mechanical treatment, gymnastics and massage. There were Red Cross treatment centres in Brighton, Holland Park and Great Portland Street in London, as well as in many Red Cross Hospitals, and the Special Orthopaedic Hospital at Shepherds Bush (run by Robert Jones) which had a special hydrological installation. The command Depots at Heaton

Park (Manchester) and at Tipperary and the First Eastern Hospital Cambridge could all provide rehabilitation facilities; there were therefore many centres outside the services which could cater for the disabled and, after the war, some of these turned to the treatment of arthritis.

After the war, interest returned to the joints and at one meeting at the RSM in 1920, F Hernaman Johnson commented that diagnoses 'even made by skilled men' sometimes proved to be wrong and that it was necessary to use 'X-rays and all the more elaborated chemical and instrumental methods as well as clinical means in making a diagnosis'. Up to this time, diagnosis was almost always a clinical matter—there being few ancillary aids. During this period as Tegner, Kersley and many others have said, the rheumatic diseases aroused little interest among general physicians—the cause of these diseases was unknown and treatment consisted of analgesics and physiotherapy, so it fell to those in charge of spas to care for the patients and stimulate research in these conditions. Lord Horder continued to deplore this lack of interest in his Heberden Oration of 1952.

In 1931 the Sections of Balneology and Climatology and that of Electrotherapy were combined into the Section of Physical Medicine—radiology was excluded. The first President was Dr FG Thompson, the Vice-presidents were Dr CB Heald, Earnest Solly and Sir Robert Stanton-Wood; the Secretaries were Dr J Sainsbury, Dr FD Howitt and Dr J Barnes-Burt. Dr FD Howitt is credited with devising the name of the section—Physical Medicine—although it had been used by the Department of the London Hospital in 1917 and he had said that although it did not appear to be a perfect name, 'it has defied all efforts to find a better one'.

The first clinical meeting of the section took place at the British Red Cross Clinic at Peto Place which had been opened the previous year for the treatment of rheumatism. The opening of this clinic brought together several interests and is considered under Rheumatology (see page 17).

Physical Therapy

In the eighteenth century, stimulation by electricity was fashionable for treating many chronic conditions. Machines were introduced from Germany early in the century and became very popular. John Wesley (1759), the founder of Methodism and part-time practitioner, used a static electrical machine for this purpose; he also wrote a home-care book on medicine *Primitive Physics*, as well as *Electricity Made Plain and Useful*. (Later Michael Farady [1791-1867] used an induction coil to produce 'faradism'.) Small departments were established at the Middlesex and St Bartholomew's Hospitals. St Bartholomew's Hospital purchased an electrical machine in 1777.

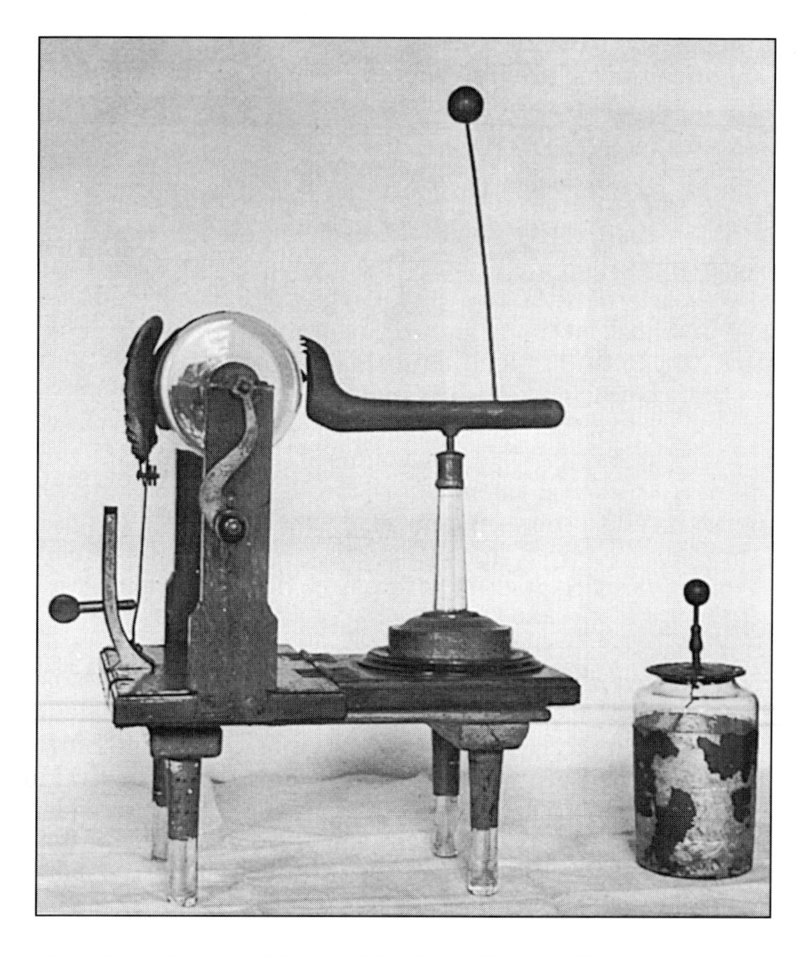

Static Electricity Machine used by John Wesley, c1747

The further development of physical medicine in hospitals was not encouraging. In 1898, at St Thomas' Hospital, it was suggested that 'a physical exercises department be added to the hospital with Mr Thursten the surgical registrar in charge, until Mr Abbot be well enough to control it'. Mr Abbot was an assistant surgeon and anatomy demonstrator. Kersley records that there was a physiotherapy department at St Bartholomew's Hospital in 1908 and at Sheffield the Edgar Allen Physical Treatment Centre was opened in 1911 but the first Physical Medicine Departments in any real sense were at the London Hospital and King's College Hospital. At the London Hospital, Dr Morton, a physicist, was employed in 1913 to investigate the effects of the passage of an electric current through the body and the Department there was started in 1917 with Sir Robert Stanton-Wood as Director. But even in 1935 the Department consisted of three separate units in different parts of the hospital: (i) massage, (ii) Tyrnauer baths (a form of hot air

(118)

(Old) leprofy
Lethargy
Lofs of appetite, of *fmell, * fpeech, * tafte
Nephritic pains
Palpitation of the heart
Pain in the back, joints, * ftomach
Rheumatifm
Rickets
Rupture
Suffocations
Surfeits (at the beginning)
Sciatica*
Scorbutic pains*
Swelling on the joints
Stone in the kidneys
Torpor of the limbs, even when the ufe of them is loft
Tetanus
Tympany
Vertigo
St. Vitus's dance
Vigilia
Varicous ulcers
The whites.

But in all cafes where the nerves are obftructed, (fuch as are thofe marked thus*) you fhould go to bed immediately after, and fweat.

'Tis often neceffary to ufe the *hot bath* a few days before you ufe the *cold.*

Wife parents fhould dip their children in cold water every morning, till they are three quarters old : and afterwards their hands and feet.

Wafhing the head every morning in cold water, prevents rheums, and cures coughs, old head-achs, and fore eyes.

WATER DRINKING generally prevents

Apoplexies, afthmas, convulfions, gout, Hyfteric fits, madnefs, palfies, ftone, trembling.

To this children fhould be ufed from their cradles.

The beft water to drink, efpecially for thofe who are much troubled with the wind, is rain-water. After it has fettled, draw it off clear into another veffel, and it will keep fweet for a long time.

ELECTRIFYING

(119)

ELECTRIFYING, in a proper manner, cures

St. Anthony's fire
Blindnefs
Blood extravafated
Bronchocele
Burns or fcalds
Coldnefs in the feet
Contraction of the limbs
Convulfions
Cramp
Deafnefs
Falling ficknefs
Feet violently difordered
Felons
Fiftula Lachrymalis
Fits
Flooding
Ganglions
Gout
Head-ach
Impofthumes
Inflammations
Involuntary motion of the eye-lids
King's Evil
Knots in the flefh
Lamenefs
Wafting
Weaknefs of the legs
Reftores bulk and fulnefs to wafted limbs
Locked jaws and joints
Leprofy
Menftrual obftructions
Ophthalmia
Pain in the ftomach
Palfy
Palpitation of the heart
Rheumatifm
Ring-worms
Sciatica
Shingles
Sinews fhrunk
Spafms
Stiff joints
Sprain, however old
Surfeit
Swellings of all forts
Sore throat
Tooth-ach
Ulcers
Wens.

Nor have I yet known one fingle inftance, wherein it has done harm ; fo that I cannot but doubt the veracity of thofe who have affirmed the contrary. Dr. *De Haen* pofitively affirms, "it can do no hurt in any cafe :" that is, unlefs the fhock be immoderately ftrong.

The beft method is to give fifty, or even a hundred fmall fhocks, each time ; but let them be fo gentle as not to terrify the patient in the leaft.

Drawing fparks removes thofe tumours on the eye-lids, called barley-corns, by exciting local inflammation, and promoting fuppuration.

Fafting-fpittle

Page from Primitive Physic, *1747, describing the use of electrification*

treatment), and (iii) electrodiagnosis. Finsen's light treatment for lupus vulgaris had been introduced at the instigation of the Princess of Wales (later Queen Alexandra) and was carried out in the Dermatology Department. Each department was supervised by a nursing sister and treatments were carried out by nurse-masseuses. Some of these nurse-masseuses eventually formed the Society of Trained Masseuses, which became the Chartered Society of Massage and Medical Gymnastics and this later again became the Chartered Society of Physiotherapy in 1943. In 1936 Sir Robert was allocated 6 beds in the hospital for the investigation and treatment of rheumatic disease; no distinction was seen between the investigation and physical treatment of these diseases.

Sir Robert Stanton-Wood studied medicine at University College Hospital and the London Hospital where he qualified. He was appointed as Consultant in Physical Medicine in 1911 at the London Hospital (the first such appointment in England). He served in World War I and after the war organised the department in the hospital. He was knighted in 1929 for his services in treating King George V during his illness. He advised the Ministry of Health on the organisation of physical medicine in the Emergency Medical Service (EMS) hospitals during World War II. He died in 1954.

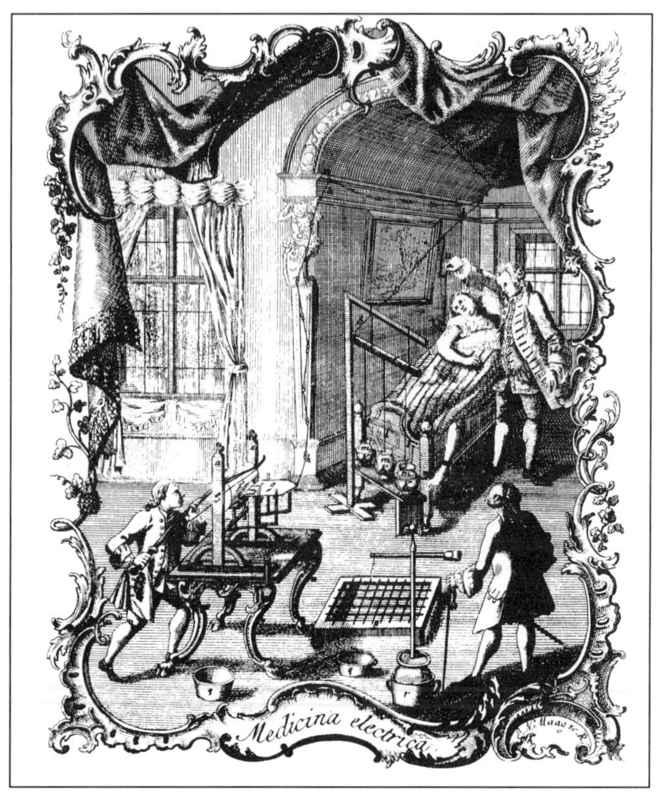

Frontispiece of Die electrische Medicin, *1766 (Wellcome Institute Library, London)*

Burt recalls that in the 1930s there were isolated physiotherapy departments in hospitals, usually called massage departments, often under the titular control of a radiologist or dermatologist. The treatments were mainly palliative, passive and empirical, although there were some active exercises prescribed. In the London Teaching Hospitals, in 1911, St Thomas' Hospital had two Swedish gymnasts who were 'treating both men and women under medical direction' but they left with the outbreak of the 1914 war and their work was delegated to two porters. At this hospital, nurses had a few lessons in massage until a training school in massage and medical gymnastics was established. In 1915, interest in the ultra-violet ray was increasing and a room was built for this, which was a forerunner of the Department of Electrotherapy, using ultra-violet light, infra-red and shortwave therapy. In 1931 Dr JB Mennell was in charge of physiotherapy, Swedish remedial exercises and massage, while Dr P Bauwens was in charge of electrotherapy. Dr Phillipe Bauwens (1901–1974) was born in Belgium and emigrated to England during World War I. At first he studied engineering but in 1918 entered St Thomas' Hospital and qualified in medicine in 1924. He was appointed as electrotherapist at St Thomas' (up until World War II,

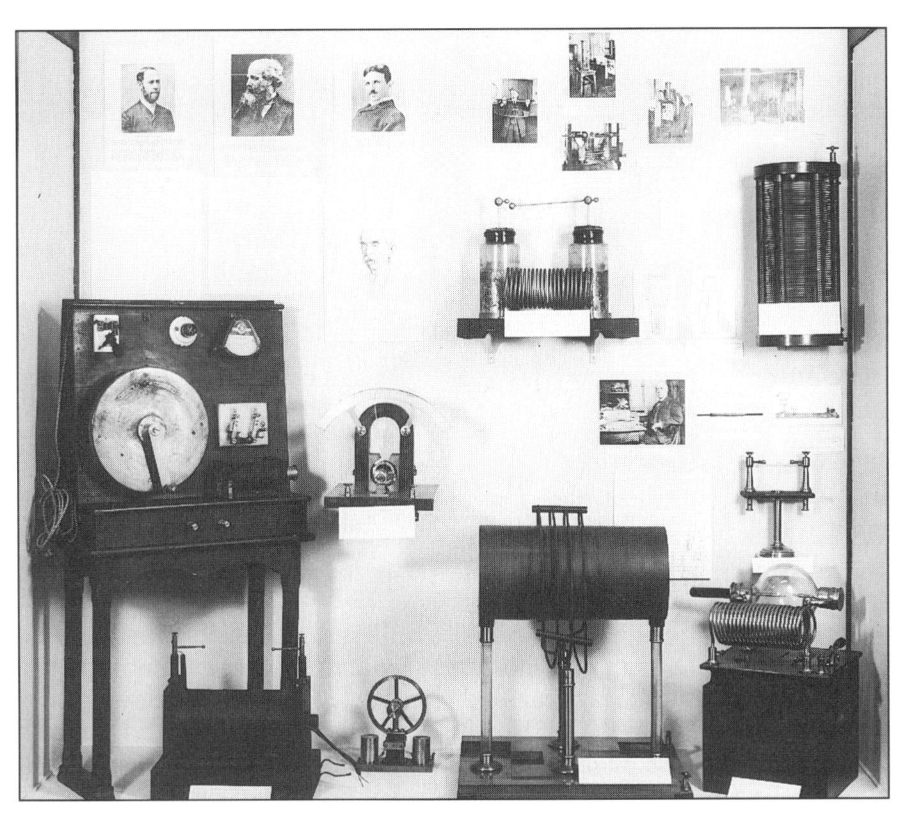

Exhibition of early electrical machines, 1892 (Wellcome Institute Library, London)

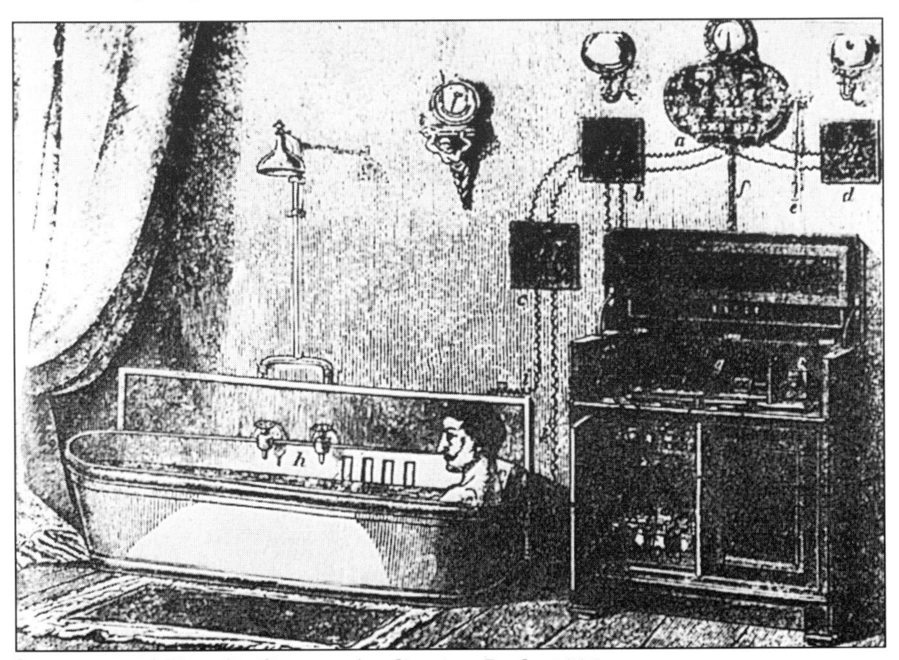

Constant and Faradic Current Application Bath, 1886

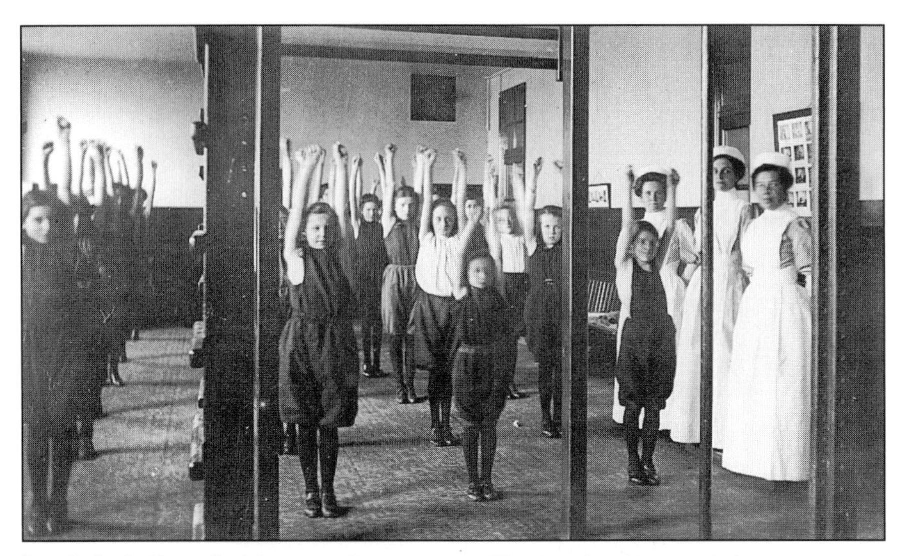

Swedish drill in the Massage Department, The London Hospital, c1910

electrotherapy was widely used) but his main contribution was the development of electrodiagnosis. He was an original member of the British Association of Physical Medicine (BAPM)—the first Secretary and President in 1956. With Dr Howitt, Lord Horder and Dr FS Cooksey, he was one of those whose influence led to the founding of the BAPM.

In that same year, in 1931, Dr CE Iredell at Guy's was recorded as being surgeon in charge of actinotherapy. Dr JF Cumberbach was

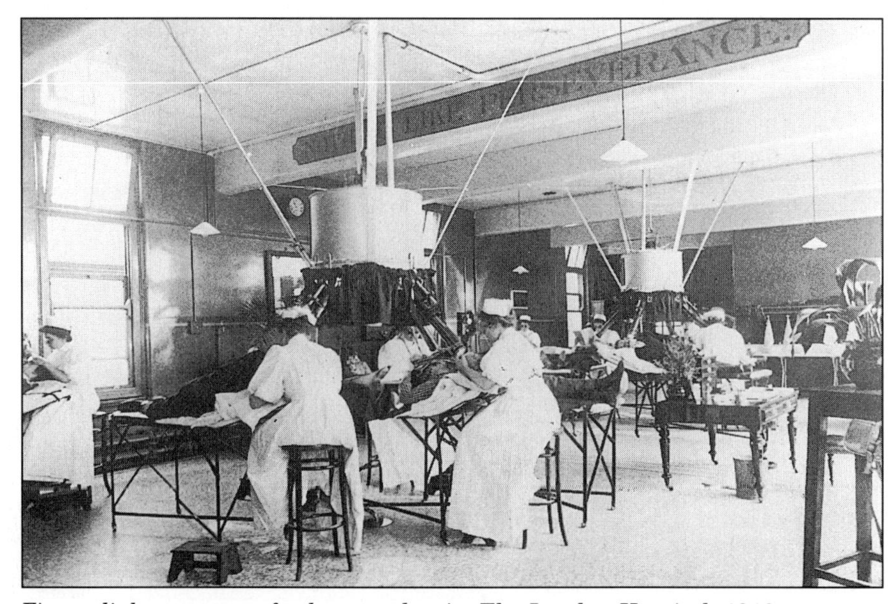

Finsen light treatment for lupus vulgaris, The London Hospital, 1910

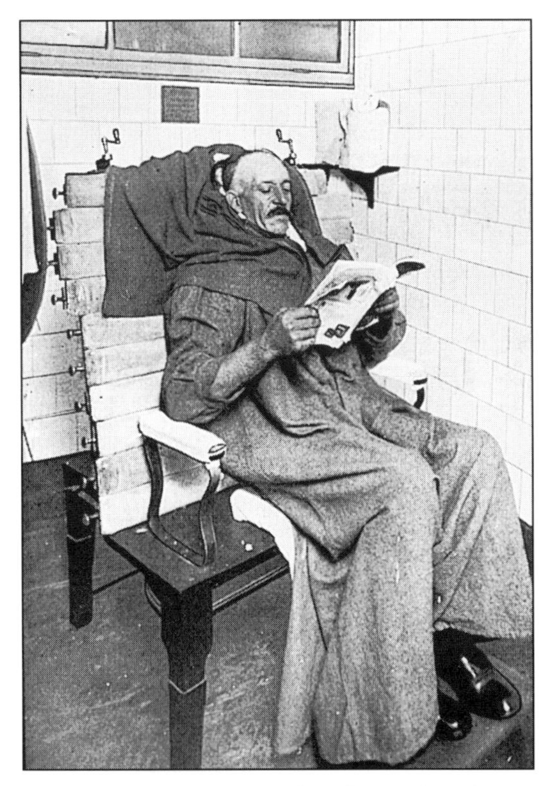

Tyrauner Bath, The London Hospital, 1909

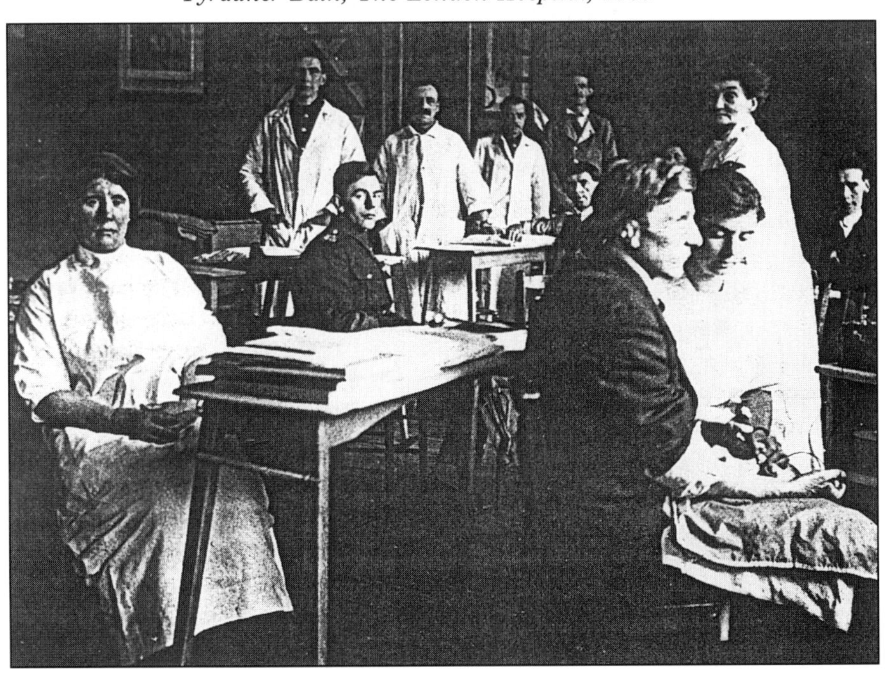

Electrical treatment during World War I

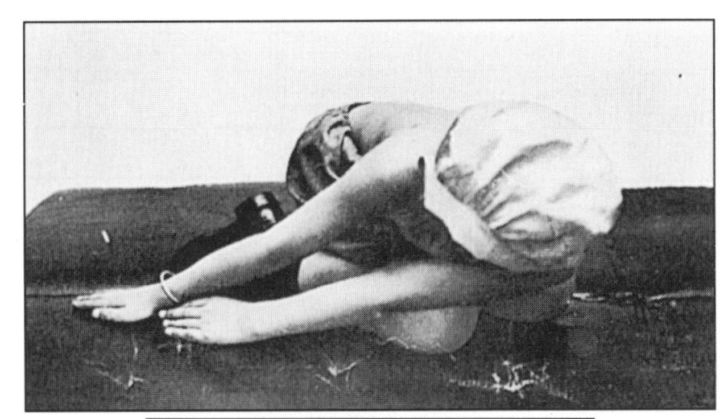

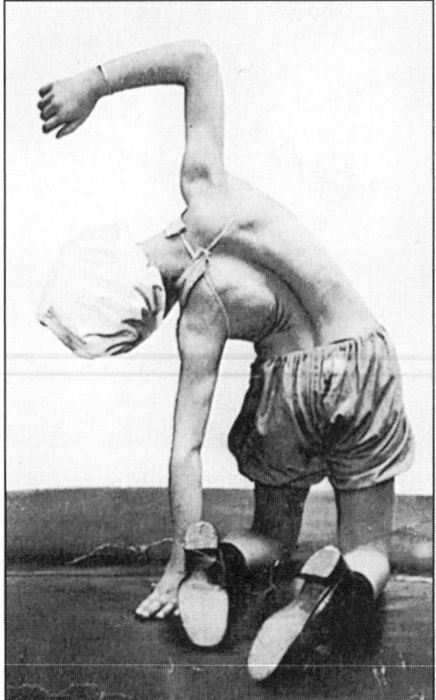

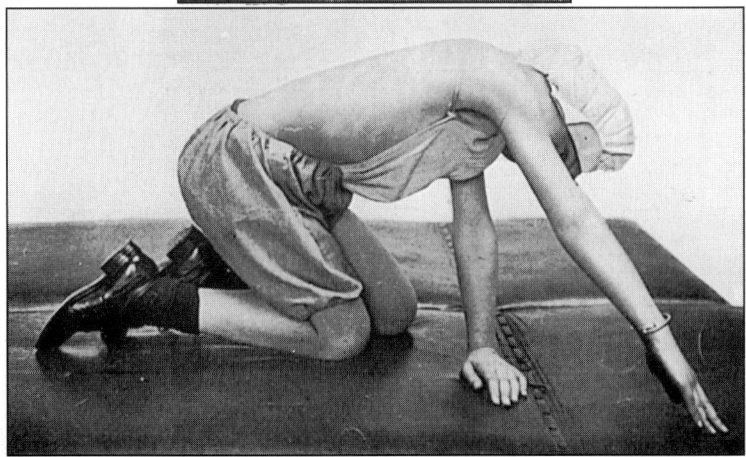

Crawling exercises, the swinging lumbar crawl, King's College Hospital, 1923 (Dr B Clayton)

in charge of the electrical department at St Bartholomew's Hospital; the Middlesex Hospital had Dr Heald and Dr Howitt in charge of the electrical department, with Dr C Fildes and Dr B Shires in the X-ray and electrotherapy department. Dr EB Clayton was in charge of physical treatment at King's College Hospital. Outside these hospitals, at the Royal Northern Hospital, in 1898 the services of trained masseuses were sought to instruct nurses in the art of 'medical rubbing'. In 1908, at this hospital, there was a new electrical department for treatment and diagnosis by electrical means (this included X-ray) which Dr Robert Knox was in charge of and it was not until 1918 that the X-ray department was separated and the title of the rest changed to physiotherapy.

At a national level, governmental matters were referred to either an orthopaedic surgeon or a radiologist until 1939, but at the beginning of World War II (on the recommendation of the British Medical Association [BMA] Group of Physical Medicine), Dr FS Cooksey was appointed Consultant Adviser to the Government.

Dr Frank Sebastian Cooksey (1891-1989) studied medicine at King's College Hospital, London and qualified there in 1929. He was the chief pioneer of modern rehabilitation medicine. He was advisor to the Government on the provision of services in EMS hospitals during World War II for which he was awarded the OBE. After the war, he had the vision to see that these services should be available to the disabled in peacetime. He advised Leonard Cheshire when the Cheshire Homes were started. He was a founder member of the BAPM and President from 1966 to 1967, as well as one of its most

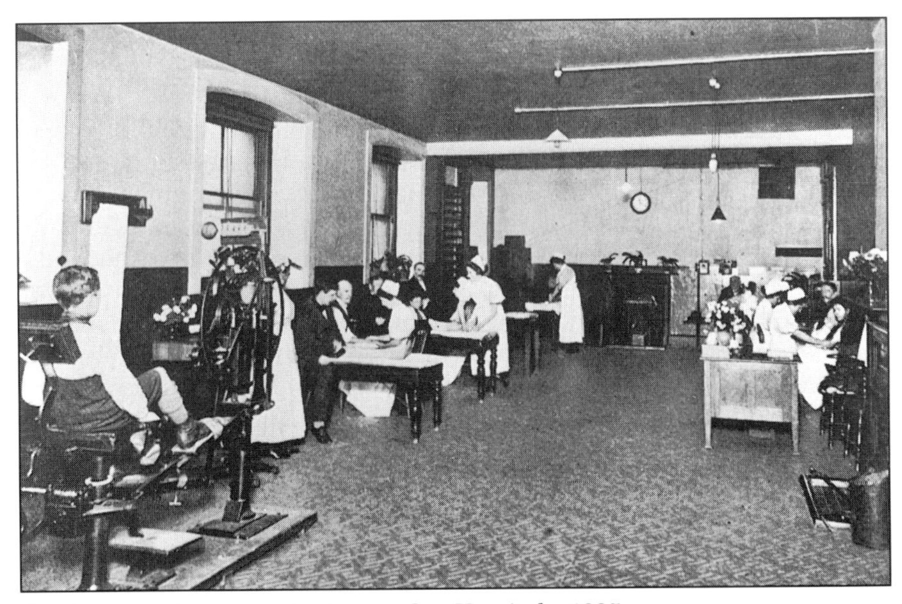

The Massage Department, The London Hospital, c1935

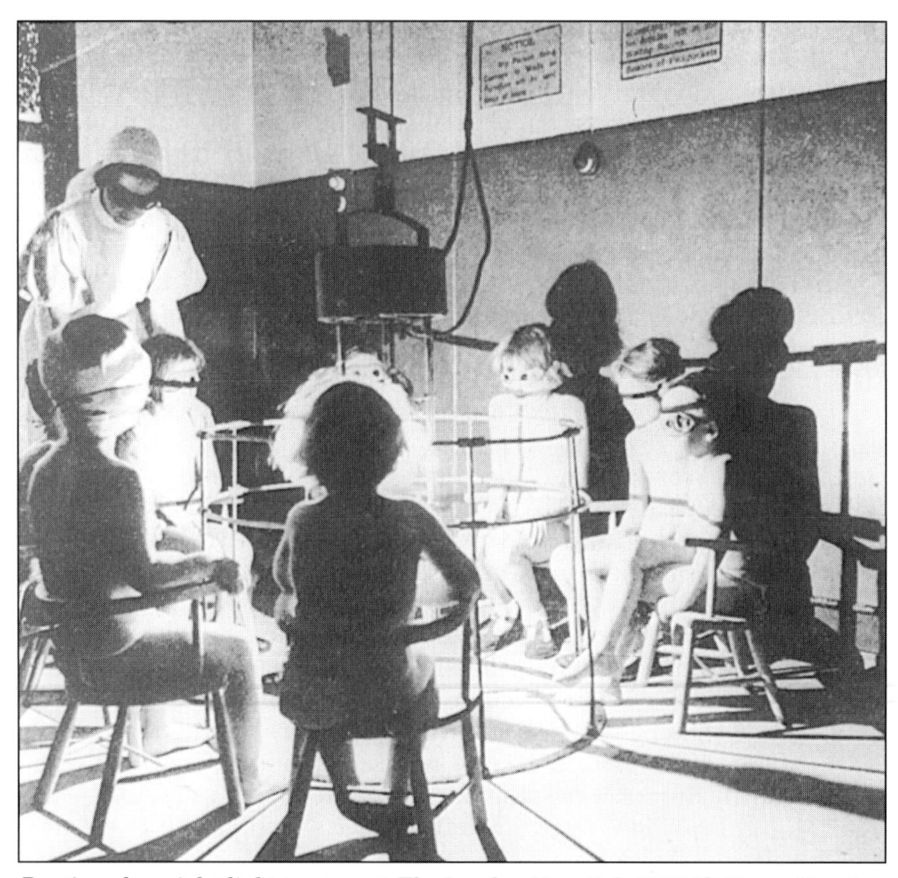

Routine ultra violet light treatment, The London Hospital c1930 (© Tower Hamlets Health Authority Archives)

active members. He was advisor to the Minister in Physical Medicine (1950–1972) and awarded the CBE in 1968. He died in 1989.

The introduction of the EMS during the war brought about an increased appreciation of physical medicine and rehabilitation. Physiotherapy departments were enlarged at all the 19 orthopaedic emergency hospitals, and Park Prewett Emergency Hospital was the first to be opened in 1939. Sir Robert Stanton-Wood, Consultant Advisor to the Government in Physical Medicine, has described the various developments in the *Medical History of the War*. Special new huts were authorised for physiotherapy and in December 1940, gymnasia were authorised. Occupational therapy was incorporated in these in 1942 with the aim of returning the sick and injured to work. Until early 1943 the facilities were only provided for service personnel, civil defence patients and air-raid casualties but later they were made more generally available which resulted in an increase in the workload. However, by 1945 inadequacies of building

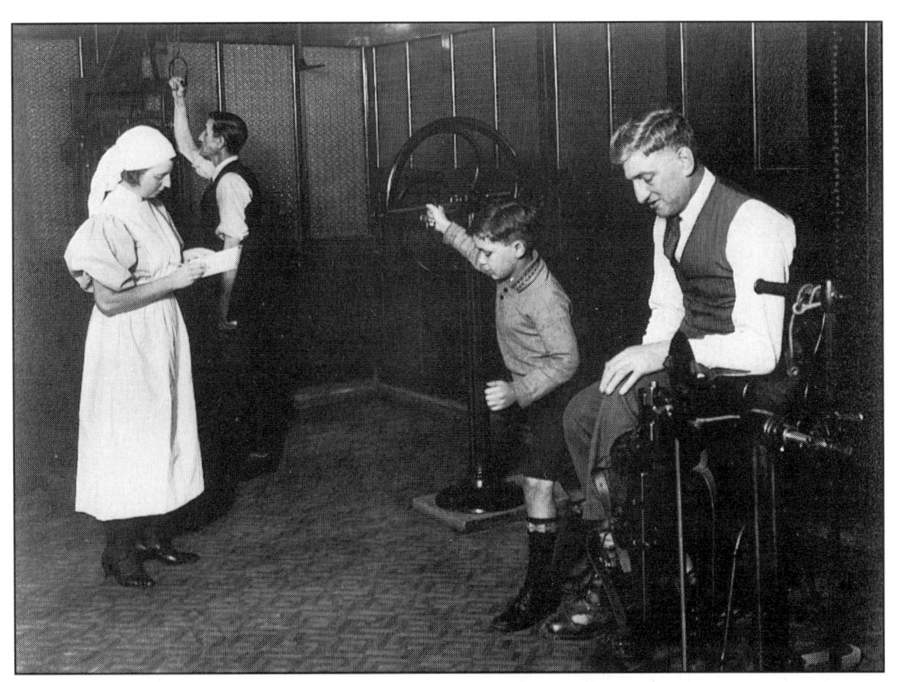

Individual exercise therapy, The London Hospital, c1937

and equipment had been largely overcome. Ultra-violet light, short-wave diathermy, heat lamps and electrodiagnostic equipment were supplied but not electromyograms and few hospitals had hydro-therapy. Some medical officers received intensive training in the techniques in use and they provided liaison with other physicians and surgeons. The training of physiotherapists was not at first recognised as an 'essential' service until 1942 when this was altered. However physiotherapists remained in short supply throughout the war. Occupational therapy which until 1939 had been almost confined to mental hospitals was now recognised as valuable for physical disease and injury. A governmental Physical Medicine Committee met in July 1940 and this later included orthopaedic surgeons and spa practitioners. A Rehabilitation Committee was also formed in 1940 but lapsed in 1943.

The Group Committee of Practitioners in Physical Medicine of the British Medical Association

In 1931, another group was started, the BMA Group of Physical Medicine Consultants. Its function was to advise the BMA on matters related to the specialty and hence influence government policy, particularly where terms and conditions of service of doctors were concerned. At the first meeting on 20 November 1931, the group was particularly concerned to stimulate research into the causes and treatment of arthritis and allied conditions and one member of the

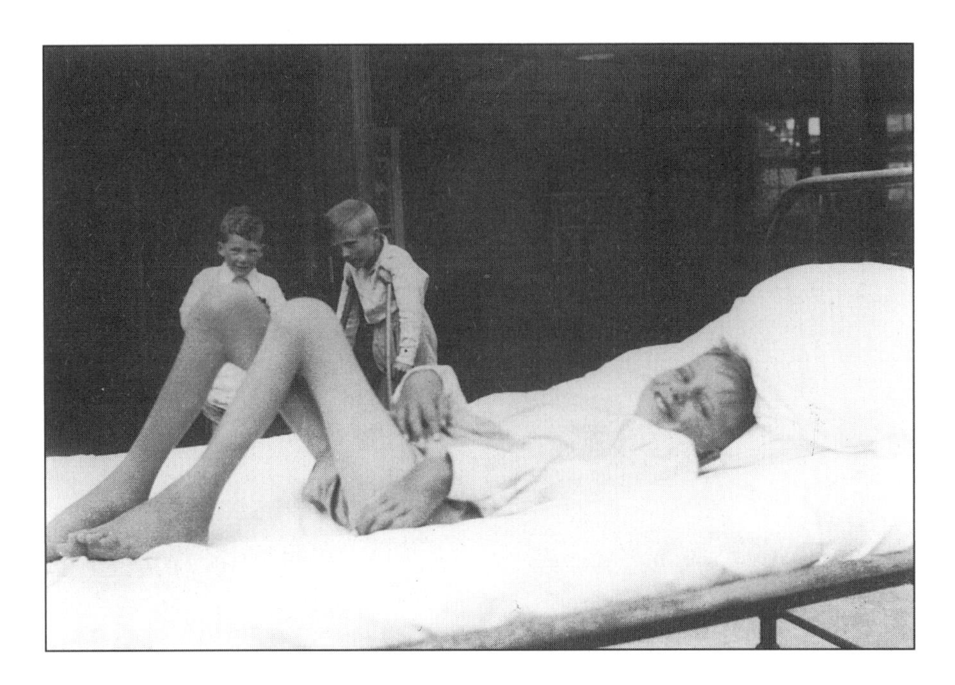

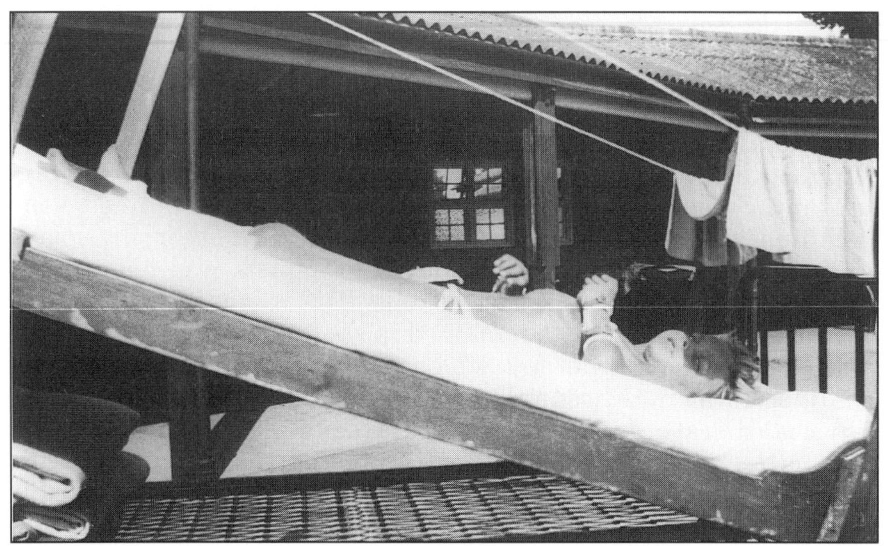

Treatment of Stills disease, before and after traction and exercises, Rowley Buster Hospital, Pyrford, later St Nicholas' and St Martin's Orthopaedic Hospital, 1935 (Wellcome Institute Library, London)

group was to be appointed to the special committee of the Royal College of Physicians (RCP) chaired by Sir Humphrey Rolleston. The scope of diseases to be studied were listed as:

(a) Atrophic arthritis
 (i) Rheumatoid arthritis

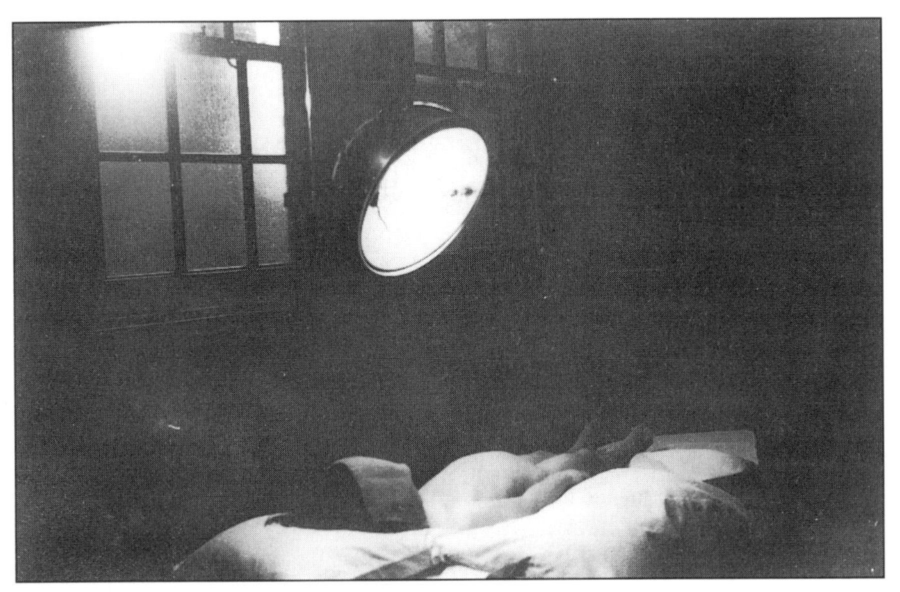

Treatment of rickets with ultra violet light, Rowley Buster Hospital, 1935

(ii) Infective
(iii) Focal
(b) Hypertrophic arthritis
(i) Osteoarthritis
(c) Fibrositis
(i) Periarticular—capsular
(ii) Muscular rheumatism—myalgia
(iii) Perineuritis—chronic non-specific neuritis

The group consisted of Dr CW Buckley, Dr CB Heald (Chairman), Dr Geoffrey Holmes, Dr F Howitt, Dr JB Mennell and Sir Robert Stanton-Wood, but others were added later. The group decided not to join the Spa Practitioners Group which had been formed by the BMA in 1927. Other subjects concerned them as well as arthritis. At that time many commercial products were advertised as containing radium and the group agreed that these were either fraudulent or very dangerous. They discussed the place of physiotherapy in medicine, the menace of quackery to physical medicine and the positions of the practitioner in physical medicine. They believed that all practitioners in physical medicine should have the MRCP or FRCS and should be full members of hospital staffs. They were concerned with undergraduate teaching of physical medicine and circulated the teaching hospitals with a questionnaire on the subject. As early as 1933 they were pressing for the establishment of a Diploma of Physical Medicine (D Phys Med), although Dr FD Howitt spoke against it. He feared that a diploma would relegate the subject to be a technical branch of medicine, whereas he felt that every effort should be made to elevate it to be a branch of general medicine. However the accepted view of the group seems to have been that the practitioner in physical medicine would be someone 'experienced primarily in general medicine but who had acquired specialised knowledge in the use and application of the physical methods employed in the practice of medicine'; there were a multiplicity of such methods of treatment in use at the time (Appendix 1). In the event in 1935 the group decided that the time was not propitious for a Diploma of Physical Medicine which was not introduced till 1944. In 1935 the group also took action to establish the name physical medicine as the accepted name for all hospital departments which up till then had worked under a variety of titles, as has already been mentioned. With the outbreak of war the group were involved in the provision of rehabilitation services in the EMS and were responsible for the appointment of Dr FS Cooksey as the adviser to the Government on the provision of rehabilitation services in civilian hospitals. Eventually they were also largely responsible for the establishment of the Dip Phys Med in 1944.

With the formation of the BAPM in 1943, the BMA group continued to act as a political platform for the specialty and was always very closely related to the Association—its successor, the British Association of Rheumatology and Rehabilitation (BARR), acquired the right to nominate a member to the group's executive council in 1979—although their importance diminished as the BAPM became more and more directly involved as a representative body for those working in the field. The fact that the chairman of the group was ex-officio a non-voting member of the Central Consultant and Specialist Committee of the BMA—later the Central Committee for Hospital Medical Services (CCHMS)—allowed the specialty a voice in professional affairs. The importance of the BMA group has been recognised more recently as being particularly important when consultant contracts were being negotiated with the DHSS. The Group changed its name to Rheumatology and Rehabilitation in 1974.

The Duchenne Society

Another group active at this time was a small number of doctors interested in electrotherapy. This group formed themselves into a dining club whose toast at each meeting was 'the Memory of Duchenne of Boulogne'. The first meeting took place at 4 Stanhope Street, London W1 on 16 November 1934. Present at this meeting were Dr WJ Turrell, Dr Howard Humphries, Dr Cumberbatch, Dr CB Heald, Dr FD Howitt and Dr P Bauwens (Secretary). As well as an interest in electrotherapy, the group agreed to combine these interests with social functions, travelling and friendly relations with other countries. Dr Heald and Dr Howitt decided not to join the society and in their place Sir Morten Smart and Dr Robinson were elected. It was decided that the membership should not exceed eight. In the next year Lord Horder joined the group. He felt it was important to separate the scientific from the pseudo-scientific as many aspects of physical medicine were open to quackery. The group discussed the possibility of forming a Physical Medicine Association and the syllabus for a possible diploma, as well as the value of electrotherapy in its various forms. Dr FS Cooksey joined the group in 1938, but with the advent of the war meetings of the Society ceased. However the spirit of the meetings was revived later in the Howitt Club.

Early Interest in Rheumatology

Meanwhile, interest in the rheumatic diseases was developing. In 1912, at the International Congress of Physiotherapy in Berlin, Dr J Van Breeman proposed the establishment of a society for scientific research into the rheumatic diseases.

Dr Jan Van Breeman (1875-1961) was the Director of the Institute of Physical Therapy in Amsterdam and later Medical Advisor and Director of the Information Bureau on Rheumatism. He has been called the father of modern rheumatology and it was he who was the driving force behind the formation of the early rheumatology societies; he stimulated European governments to become interested in the subject. He was secretary of the International League and editor of the *Acta Rheumatologue*. There are many papers by him on the aetiology of rheumatoid arthritis in the journals at that time. He died in 1961.

World War I prevented further development, but in 1921 Dr Robert Fortescue Fox founded the International Society of Medical Hydrology (ISMH) at a meeting at the RSM in London—the Society started a journal, the *Archives of Medical Hydrology*, which ran from 1925 to 1939 with a few numbers in 1948.

Dr Robert Fortescue Fox qualified at the London Hospital in 1883. At first, he was in practice at the spa in Strathpeffer but then settled in London. He was an active member of La Ligue Internationale Contre le Rheumatisme, as well as a foundation member of the Empire Rheumatism Council (ERC). He was co-author with Dr J Van Breeman of *The Causation and Treatment of Rheumatism* and wrote extensively on rheumatism and medical hydrology. He died in 1939.

In 1925, at the instigation of Dr Van Breeman, a special sub-committee of the ISMH was formed to consider the prevention and treatment of rheumatic disease (Dr J Alison Glover had produced his report on the incidence of the rheumatic diseases in 1924). In the same year (1925) it was suggested that there should be a British Committee on Rheumatism (one report says that there was a meeting of this committee on 25 June 1925) but it seems there was some delay in forming the full committee which probably did not meet until

1 July 1926. Representation was a wide one—there were representatives from the London County Council, the Federated Trades Unions, the National Conference of Friendly Societies, the BMA Insurance Acts Committee, the Ministry of Health (Dr J Alison Glover), the Balneology section of the RSM (Dr MB Ray), the ISMH (Dr F Fox and Dr EP Poulton), the British Spa Federation (Dr CW Buckley, Dr JB Burt from Buxton, Dr V Coates from Bath, Dr W Edgecombe, Dr G Holmes, Dr K Pringle and Dr AP Friel from Harrogate, and Dr LJ Llewellyn from London). There was also an Advisory Committee which included Lord Dawson of Penn, Sir Humphrey Rolleston, Sir Archibald Garrod, Sir William Hale-White, Dr L Hill, Professor TSP Strangeways and Sir Thomas Horder who joined the panel later. Dr Fortescue Fox was the Chairman of the main Committee and Dr MB Ray was the Secretary. The Committee paid visits to the physical treatment centres in Germany which led to their recommendations for the setting up of the Peto Place Red Cross Clinic for the treatment of rheumatism (to be considered later, see page 19).

On 27 November 1925, a joint meeting between the Section of Balneology and Climatology of the RSM and the ISMH was held at 1 Wimpole Street, London, and Sir George Newman put forward his ideas for a satisfactory rheumatological service. He proposed that there should be: (1) out-patient clinics with physical treatment; (2) arthritic units preferably related to teaching hospitals for research and orthopaedic liaison; and (3) spa hospitals for treatment of suitable cases. These ideas were further developed by Dr J Alison Glover in 1926 at a meeting of the Dutch Committee on Chronic Rheumatism in Amsterdam and again by Sir George Newman at a conference in Bath in May 1928 and in the same year, Dr J Alison Glover issued his second report on the chronic rheumatic diseases.

Sir George Newman (1870-1948) qualified in medicine in 1891 from the University of Edinburgh and Kings College, London. He was Medical Officer of Health for Finsbury from 1900-1907, then Chief Medical Officer at the Board of Education until 1919 and subsequently Chief Medical Officer of the Ministry of Health until his retirement in 1935. Apart from his support for rheumatology, he wrote extensively on other subjects—the prevention of tuberculosis, medical education, leprosy, and infant mortality were some of the subjects covered. The London School of Hygiene and Tropical Medicine and The Royal Post-graduate Medical School owe their existence to him.

Dr James Alison Glover OBE (1870-1963) qualified in 1901 at Guy's Hospital. He was a Medical Officer in the Ministry of Health and the official representative on early rheumatology committees. It was his reports on chronic rheumatic diseases of 1924 and 1928 which brought the subject to official notice in England. He wrote extensively and particularly on cerebrospinal meningitis.

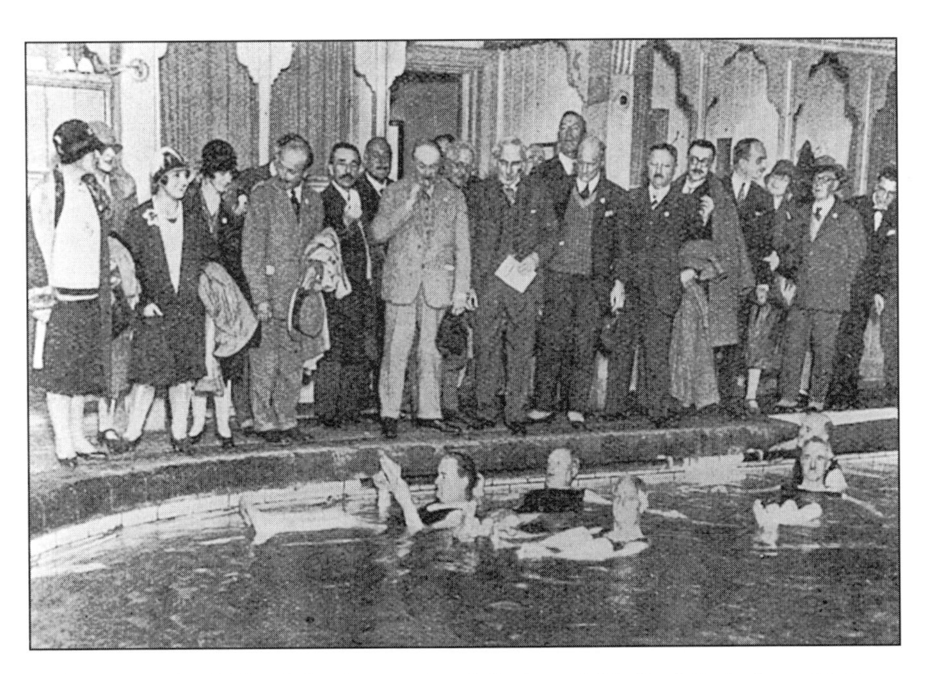

Delegates at the AGM of the International Society of Medical Hydrology, 1928, at St Andrew's bath, Droitwich

In October 1928, the Rheumatology Committee of the ISMH (with the parent body—the ISMH) held its Annual General Meeting (AGM) in England and visited London, Harrogate, Buxton, Droitwich and Bath. It was at this meeting at Buxton that the International Committee on Rheumatology constituted itself as La Ligue Internationale Contre le Rhumatisme—a journal was produced, *The Acta Rheumatalogica*, which ran from 1929 to 1939. The first full meeting of La Ligue took place in Budapest in October 1929.

The Red Cross Clinic for the Treatment of Rheumatism

A sub-committee of the British Committee on Rheumatism produced a memorandum in 1927 reported in the *British Medical Journal (BMJ)* defining the problem of rheumatism. They defined three types: (1) acute forms; (2) subacute forms; and (3) mechanical impediments. They called for a rheumatic clinic to deal with patients fit to walk or be brought to it but who did not need in-patient treatment. The suggestion that sufferers might be transferred to a spa was thought to involve too much expense. The plans for such a unit were laid before a committee appointed by the Red Cross of which Sir Arthur Stanley was Chairman and they became the sponsors of the British Red Cross Clinic at Peto Place for the treatment of rheumatism. It was opened in 1930 by Queen Mary. Boyle (1972) has given an account of the building and the opening ceremony. The building was constructed in 1827 as a diorama, giving people a panoramic view

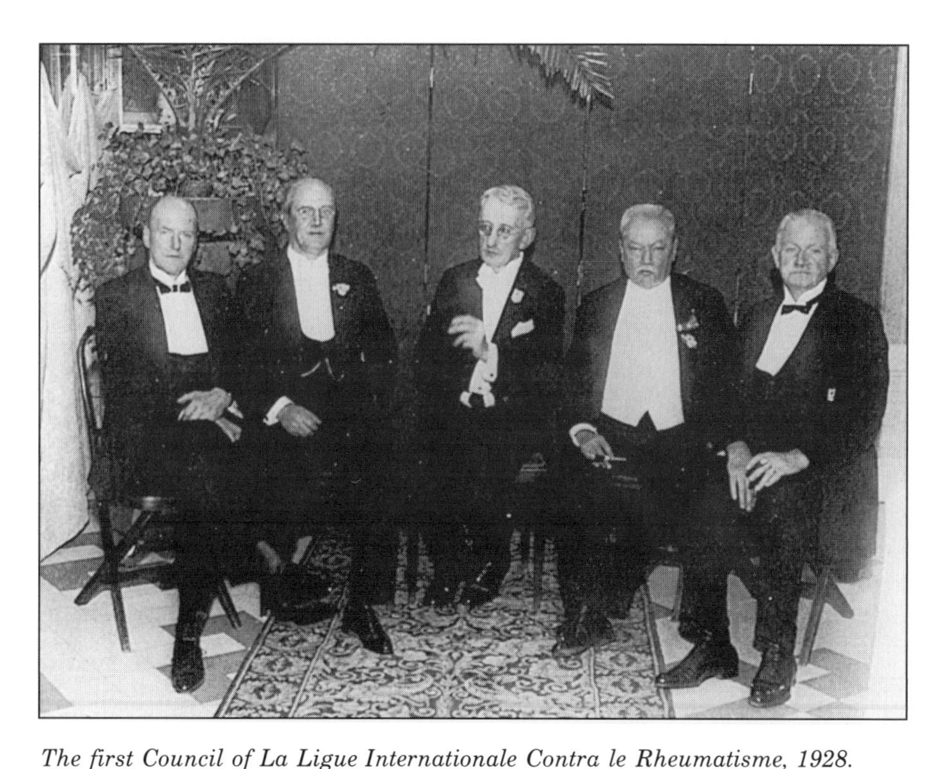

The first Council of La Ligue Internationale Contra le Rheumatisme, 1928.

Dr J van Breeman, Professor Dr Z Vamossy, Dr R Fortescue Fox, Dr Barona A von Koranyi, Professor Dr Dietrich

of London but was then converted into a Baptist chapel by a certain Mr Martin Peto (his name is perpetuated in the name of the alley way). Many dignitaries attended the opening ceremony—both the Mayor of St Pancras and the Mayor of St Marylebone attended as the clinic lay between the two boroughs, the front door opening into one borough and the back door into the other. A single treatment cost 3s or a course of not less than eight treatments, 25s. The top floor was reserved for private patients. The treatments consisted of '(1) heat, cold, movement in water vapour and hot air locally and generally; (2) manipulation and exercises alone or in combinations with heat, by hand or by douches or whirling water; (3) radiation—as heat, light, visible and invisible (ultraviolet and infra-red) from arc or mercury vapour and other lamps; and (4) electricity—as constant current to resolve exudate and promote nutrition; as interrupted current to cause movement of muscle fibres; and as high frequency current (diathermy) to raise the temperature of deep-seated parts'. The Red Cross Society issued a pamphlet outlining the needs of such a clinic which could be applied to clinics in the future.

The honorary visiting physicians who treated the patients were originally five in number—Dr MB Ray, Dr FD Howitt, Dr CB Heald,

NOTED CHAPEL
CONVERTED BY
RED CROSS.

FIRST OF ITS KIND
IN COUNTRY.

LONDON SPA.

WONDER BATHS FOR
RHEUMATIC PATIENTS

When the Queen opens next Tuesday the new rheumatism clinic founded by the British Red Cross at Regent's Park, she will press a valve that fills with hot salt water the large bathing-pool in the main hall.

This will be the signal for the opening to the public of the first rheumatism clinic to be established in this country.

The Red Cross Clinic for the Treatment of Rheumatism, Peto Place, Daily Chronicle, *1930*

Dr BS Nisse and Dr WSC Copeman. Dr Francis Bach was medical registrar. These five physicians formed the Committee for the Study and Investigation of Rheumatism in 1936 and the following year the name was changed to 'The Heberden Society' of which Dr FD Howitt was the first President, while the next two were Dr MB Ray and Dr CB Heald, both prominent members of the first council of BAPM. At a later date with the introduction of the National Health Service (NHS) it did not seem proper for the clinic at Peto Place to remain financed by the Red Cross when treatment became a national responsibility. This therefore passed to the Middlesex Hospital and the clinic was renamed the Arthur Stanley Institute. In later years it seemed rational to amalgamate the Physical Medicine Department of the Hospital and the Institute and a new building was erected—Arthur Stanley House. Money was provided by the Nuffield Foundation and the Arthritis and Rheumatism Council, allowing not only a clinical department to be formed but a Department of Rheumatological Research and a Department of Immunology to be incorporated. The building was opened by Her Majesty Queen Elizabeth in 1972.

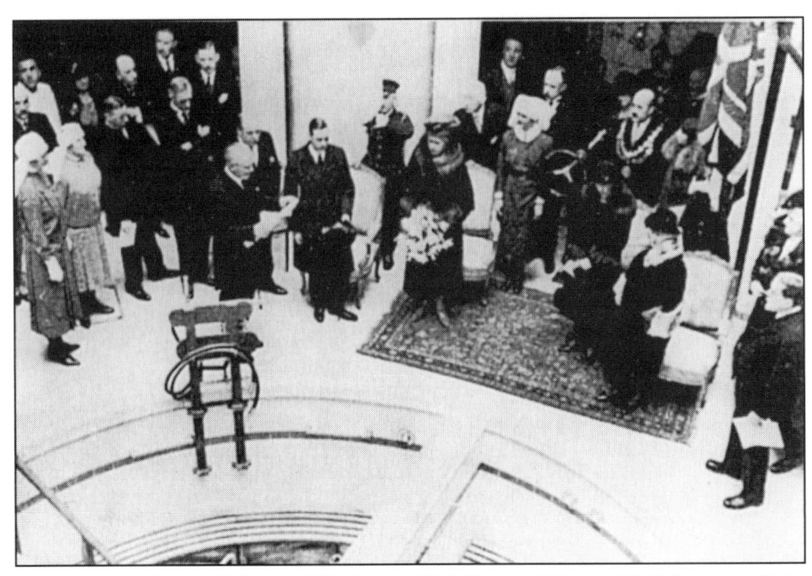

Opening of the Red Cross Clinic by HM Queen Mary, 25 February 1930 (Central News Ltd)

Mr FC Davies (Secretary), The Minister of Health, Sir Arthur Stanley, General Champain, HRH The Duke of York, HM The Queen, Sir Otto Beit, Dr Neligan (Medical Superintendent), Miss MacAllister (Sister-in-Charge), Mayor of St Marylebone, HRH Princess Mary, Princess Louise, Lady Airtie, Sir Edward Stewart

However, during this time other developments were taking place in the field of rheumatology. The British Committee on Rheumatism was dissolved in 1929 in favour of a National Campaign against Rheumatism of which Lord Horder was Chairman and Dr MB Ray was Secretary, but according to Copeman (1935) the work was frustrated, mainly because of the world depression until 1932 when at a meeting of the International Committee in Paris, Britain was urged to form a permanent body to explore the field of rheumatism. As a result an *ad hoc* committee was set up in July 1933 with Sir Humphrey Rolleston as Chairman, even though doubts were expressed at the RCP whether the time was opportune for such a committee. (The medical profession still seemed reluctant to treat the subject seriously.) However, the *ad hoc* committee remained in being but not as an official committee of the RCP. (This presumably was a continuation of the committee appointed by the BMA in 1931.) The committee included Dr WSC Copeman, Dr J Alison Glover, Dr MH Gordon, Professor AJ Hall, Dr G Holmes, Dr AA Mancrieff, Dr GH Oriel, Dr EP Poulton, Sir Humphrey Rolleston, Dr EC Warners, Sir William Willcox and Sir Thomas Horder replaced Professor AJ Hall later. This committee consisted of all medical members. Further, as a result of the advice of this special committee, the RCP in 1936 recommended that the committee should act as

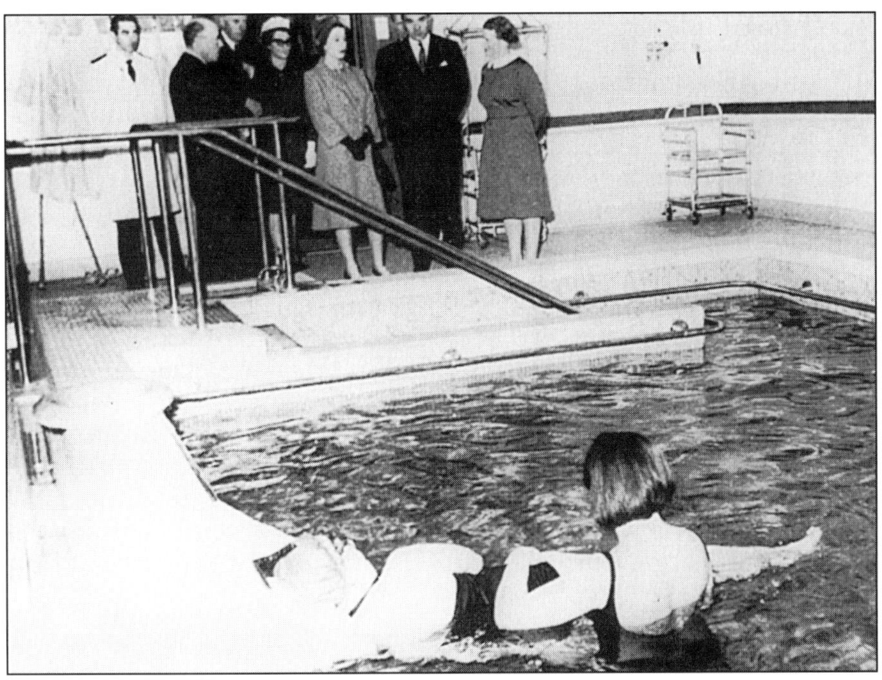

Opening of the Arthur Stanley Institute, 1970

Brigadier Hardy-Roberts, HM Queen Elizabeth II, Dr AC Boyle, Miss Duffield

a Scientific Advisory Committee to advise on a campaign against rheumatism. This resulted in the formation of the ERC, which consisted of both lay and medical members; Lord Horder was the Chairman. The Scientific Advisory Committee to the council now consisted of 30 medical members with Dr MN Gordon as Chairman, and Lord Horder and Dr WSC Copeman (Secretary) of the main council as ex-officio members. The membership included Dr FJ Bach, Dr G Holmes, Dr GD Kersley, Dr WS Tegner, Sir Robert Stanton Wood and Dr MB Ray—all later involved in the inauguration of the BAPM. The ERC became the Arthritis and Rheumatism Council (ARC) in 1964.

Dr Matthew Burrow Ray (DSO, OBE, MD, MRCP) qualified at Edinburgh University in 1893. He served in World War I and was awarded the DSO in 1917. His early medical career was spent in Harrogate where he was Honorary Surgeon to Harrogate Infirmary. With his experience in medical hydrology, he came to London and was founder member of the staff of the British Red Cross Clinic at Peto Place. He was the second President of the Heberden Society (1937) and was a member of many of the early committees on rheumatology and Secretary of the National Campaign against Rheumatism (1929). He was a founder member of the BAPM and its first Treasurer, and was the first BAPM Editor of the *British*

Journal of Physical Medicine in 1946. He was awarded the OBE in 1945. He died in 1950.

Specific rheumatology units were opened at the West London Hospital with Dr WSC Copeman in charge in 1938 and at St Stephen's Hospital in the previous year, but physical treatment was regarded as necessary at some stage in every type of arthritis and hydrological treatment, as at a spa, an invaluable adjunct (J Alison Glover, 1928).

Electrodiagnosis

In the nineteenth century, there had developed an interest in the electrical properties of the neuro-muscular system. Duchenne had observed the difference in galvanic/faradic responses in denervated muscle and it was Erb who later named this the 'Reaction of Degeneration (RD)'. At that time the most concern was with the changes in Rheobase and Chronaxi and it was not until the early twentieth century that these features were combined in the Intensity/Duration Curve (I/T curve). This curve was plotted at first

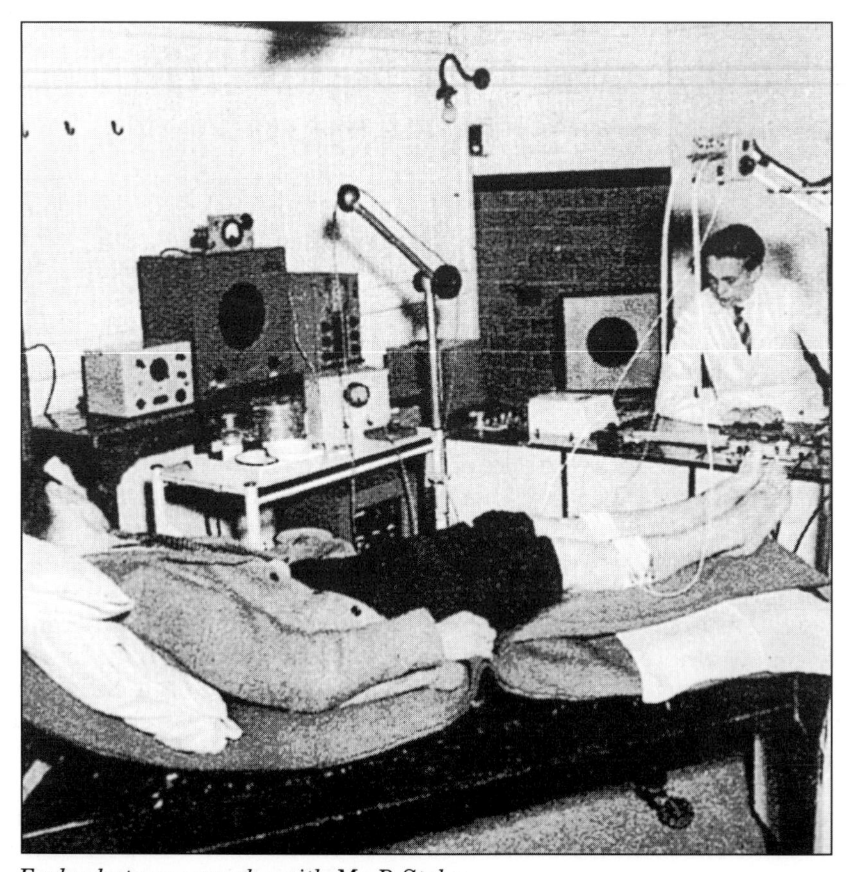

Early electromyography with Mr P Styles

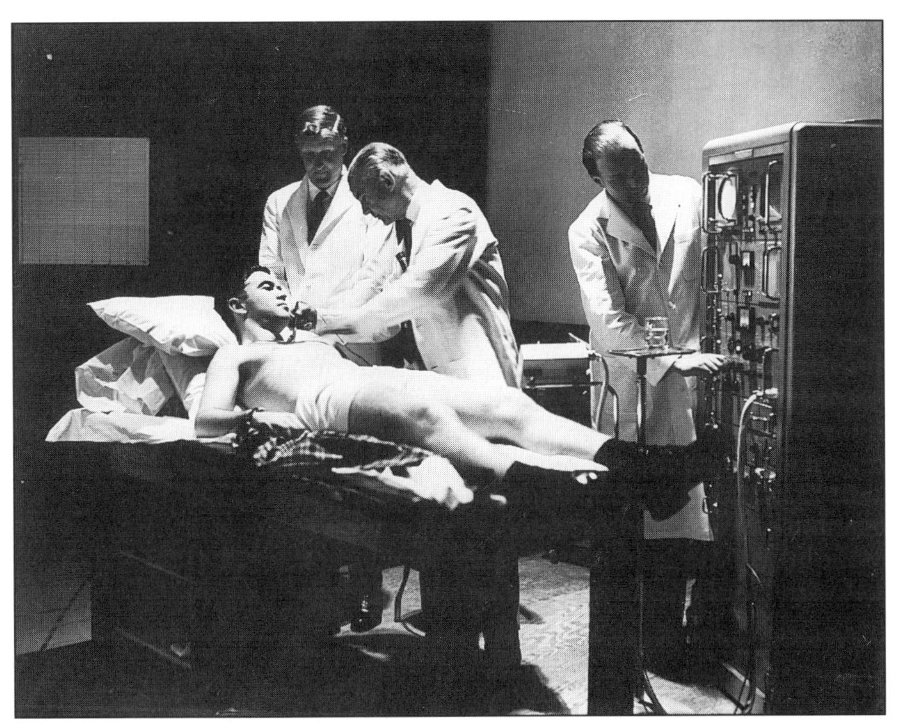

Electrodiagnosis, St Thomas' Hospital, London, c1950

Dr AT Richardson, Dr P Bauwens, Mr P Styles

with the Ritchie-Sneath Instrument a constant voltage machine, but later Dr Bauwens introduced a constant current machine which was more accurate and easy to use. This was later (1960) simplified by Mr Peter Styles to give the main significant points on this curve, although there was a movement later to reintroduce the constant voltage machine. Electromyography (EMG) did not develop until the twentieth century when Adrian and Bronk in 1929 used a concentric needle electrode to record impulses from the triceps of man. Previously, surface electrodes had been used by Richter (1927) and Wochholder (1923) using two needle electrodes separated by 2 cm. It then became possible to differentiate the main clinical entities by EMG, and it was Weddell *et al.* (1949) who first published the electromyographic findings in normal and pathological conditions in a large series of patients. Although these tests were primarily of neurological concern, the development of the instruments required electronic expertise (Buller AJ and Styles P, 1952) and this was supplied at St Thomas' Hospital in the Department of Physical Medicine under the direction of Dr P Bauwens. The Physical Medicine Section of the RAF at Chessington had also been carrying out research in this field. Mr Peter Styles, an electronic engineer from the army, joined the team at St Thomas' after the war and liaison with the Oxford laboratory run by Dr Weddell was established as well as with the RAF so that by 1950, Bauwens and Richardson could describe a fairly standardised routine for investigating neuro-muscular diseases. Regular teaching sessions were held and the physical medicine consultant became the main provider of electrodiagnosis in many hospitals.

Early Rehabilitation

Until after the 1939–1945 war, rehabilitation had been largely promoted by the armed services and seen as a way of getting servicemen back into action; it had been an orthopaedic concern. Wittaker states that there was really no rehabilitation during the Crimean War but 'if the weather was clement, convalescents would be frequently marched about'. Perhaps the first effort at rehabilitation was the establishment of the Lord Roberts Workshops for soldiers of the Boer War. In the 1914–1918 war, convalescent depots were started in the Army largely with the idea of emptying the hospitals although the Kings Lancashire Military Convalescent Hospital at Blackpool seems to have provided a wide range of therapeutic procedures. The brochure of the hospital in 1917 records that the hospital had a gymnasium for physical exercises of all types: an electromassage and hydrotherapy department with whirlpool baths. 'Shell shock patients were treated by passing electricity through the brain'. Electro-convulsive therapy (ECT) was not used in England until 1933. There was a hot exercise room: 'exercises were done both with and without machines and there were heat and light baths to break down adhesions'. In addition, Dr TB Nichols in 1937 spoke of the value of graduated exercises under medical supervision to hasten convalescence and retrain soldiers. He also emphasised the value of sea-bathing and swimming pool therapy in assisting this process and it is clear that outside the services, the spas and the Red Cross were providing extensive rehabilitation facilities as already discussed.

However, the pioneering work in rehabilitation is attributed to Sir Robert Jones. Robert Jones (1857–1933) qualified in medicine in 1878 from the Liverpool School of Medicine. He was assistant surgeon at the Stanley Hospital, Liverpool and surgeon at the Royal Southern Hospital. He became interested in 'prevention and correction of deformities in children' (orthopaedics) and in 1900 contributed to the opening of the childrens' hospital at Heswell. He and Dame Agnes Hunt were associated with the Baschurch House at Oswestry which provided home care for 'crippled children' in 1909. Sir Pandrill Varmier-Jones had founded the Papworth Village Settlement for tuberculosis sufferers but the main contribution to rehabilitation was Sir Robert's work at the Military Orthopaedic Hospital in Shepherds Bush during the 1914–1918 war. He had started Alder Hey Hospital for the Wounded in 1915, and when the

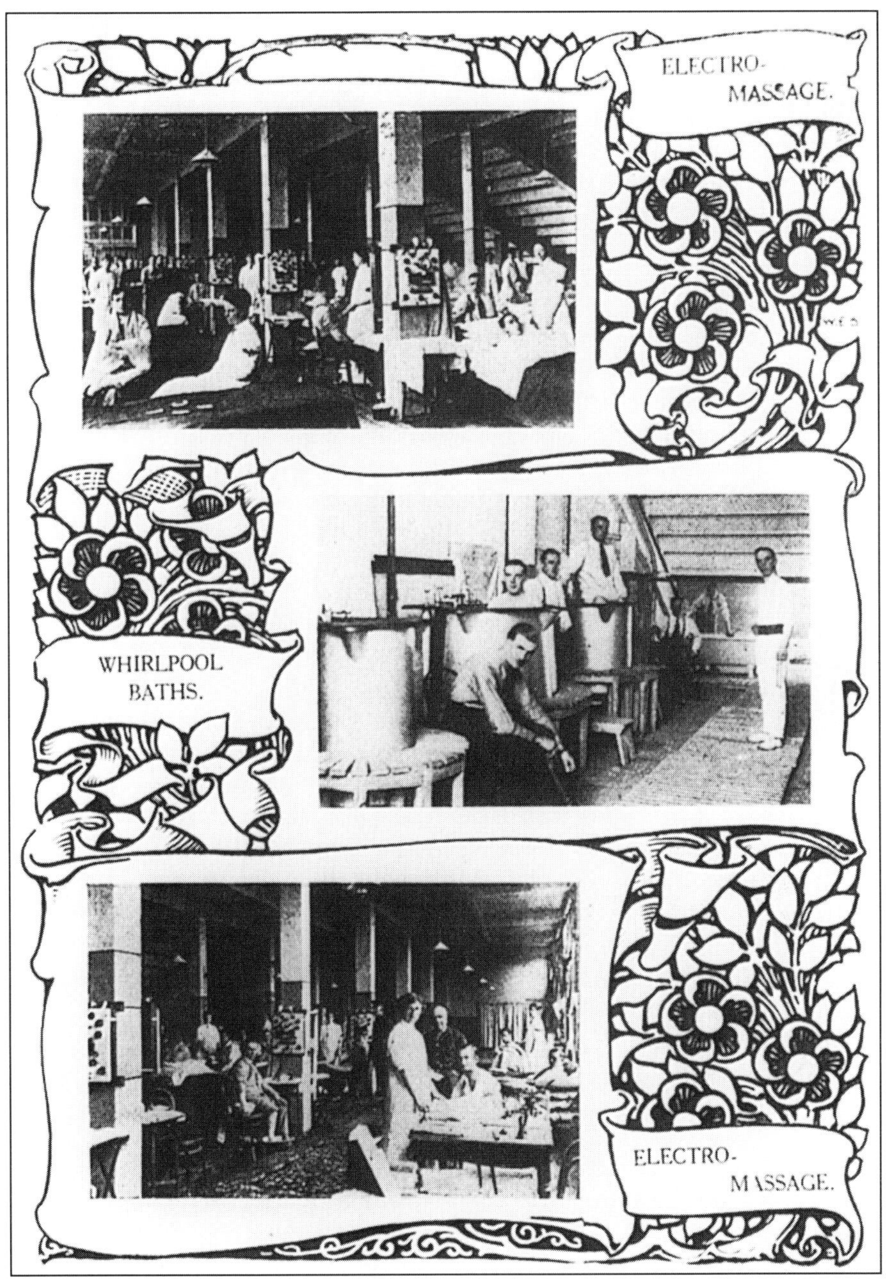

Treatments available at the King's Lancashire Military Convalescent Hospital, Blackpool, 1917 (Wellcome Institute, London)

Hammersmith workhouse was taken over by the War Office with a grant from the Red Cross, Robert Jones developed a 'Curative Workshop' there which was opened on 1 March 1916. Wounded soldiers often received massage and electrical treatment with monotonous exercises but his workshop provided useful and productive work to hasten recovery. For those to be discharged from the Army, it provided a bridge to civilian life. Robert Jones was knighted in 1917. The Ministry of Pensions took over the unit in 1919 (the Red Cross bequeathed the equipment to the Ministry), but the unit was closed in 1925 and the pioneer work was not followed up by others, although during the war through His Majesty King Manoell of Portugal, who was the Red Cross representative, rehabilitation facilities were available at other Red Cross Hospitals. Sir Robert Jones and Mr Girdlestone were associated with the Committee for the Care of Cripples under the auspices of the British Red Cross in 1919 and there was a Red Cross clinic for the physical treatment of officers in Great Portland Street but this seems to have been given up after the war. However, most other long-term care of the disabled was in the hands of voluntary charitable organisations with specific groups such as the blind, the deaf and the crippled particularly looked after. There were establishments such as St Loyes College at Exeter, Queen Elizabeth's Foundation for the Disabled at Leatherhead and Enham Village Settlements at Andover.

Physical Fitness

Between the wars, Sir George Newman's reports of 1919 and 1926 on the value of physical training gymnastics and organised games in the open air seemed to have gone largely unheeded, for their value in the 1914-1918 war had been appreciated at the time and he had recommended that every child should have daily organised physical exercise. All the same, the standard of physical fitness in recruits to the army was found to be terribly poor. Because of this, a physical training centre was opened at Aldershot in 1937 and others were opened at the outbreak of war.

As in the past, the outbreak of the 1939 war resulted in the increased concern with both rehabilitation and physical fitness, and both the Army and RAF were quick to appreciate this. The Navy followed later.

The Army

In 1940 Dr Frank Howitt was asked by the Government to report on the rehabilitation being carried out at a military convalescent unit at the Royal Bath Hospital in Harrogate in the care of an orthopaedic surgeon. As a result of this report, the principles in use there were extended to all convalescent depots and Dr Howitt was appointed Consultant in Physical Medicine to the Army with the rank of Brigadier.

He recruited a team of consultants in Physical Medicine, Dr J Patterson, Dr GD Kersley, Dr H Turney, Dr WS Tegner, Dr JJR Duthie, Dr A Wesson and Dr P Davies. These physicians were promoted to the rank of Major to set up Rehabilitation Units at

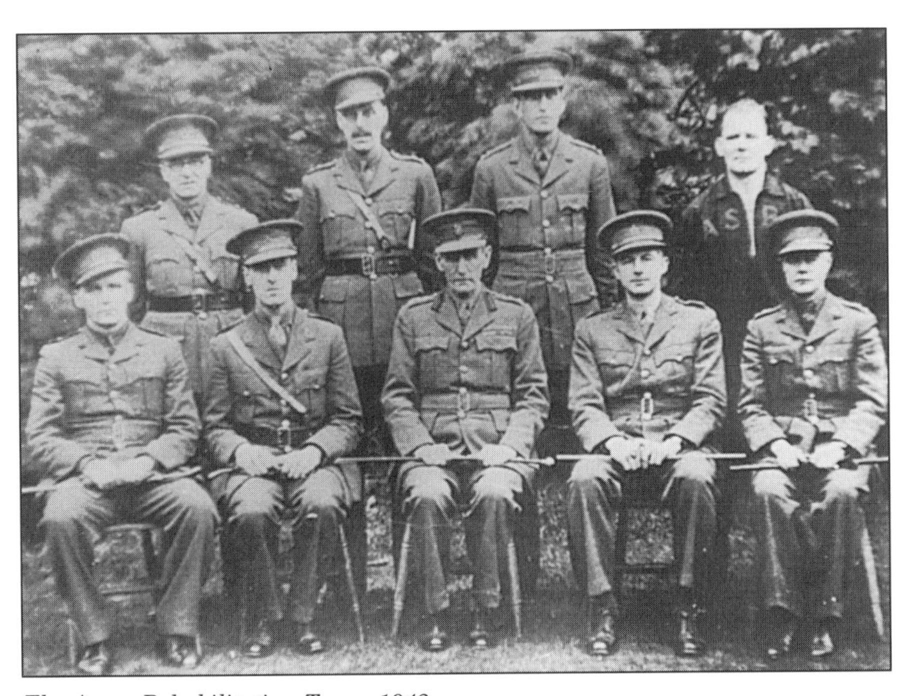

The Army Rehabilitation Team, 1942

Majors Patterson, Tegner, Turney and Mr Slade, Majors Duthie, Kersley, Col Dyer, Majors Davies and Wesson

all convalescent depots at home and abroad. The emphasis at the centres was on progressive exercises in graded classes mixed with games and Kersley has given a graphic account of his experiences as a Physical Medicine Adviser in the Army in his book *The Three Rs.* Dr Doris Baker joined the team from the ATS.

The British Red Cross had various convalescent hospitals particularly at Middleton Park but these units were thought to be too civilian orientated and army personnel were posted to them to improve discipline.

The RAF

Rehabilitation in the RAF started in 1940 under the leadership of Sir Reginald Watson-Jones, Sir Henry Osmond-Clark and Group Captain JBS O'Malley and was mainly directed at orthopaedic patients. The first unit (opened in the Palace Hotel Torquay) was for officers but this building suffered bomb damage and the unit was moved inland. The convalescent depot at Blackpool was also devoted to rehabilitation and a unit was opened at Loughborough College under the direction of Group Captain JBS O'Malley, CBE. In all, there were six centres open during the war. The routine of treatment consisted of formal exercises, remedial games, physiotherapy, occupational therapy with walks

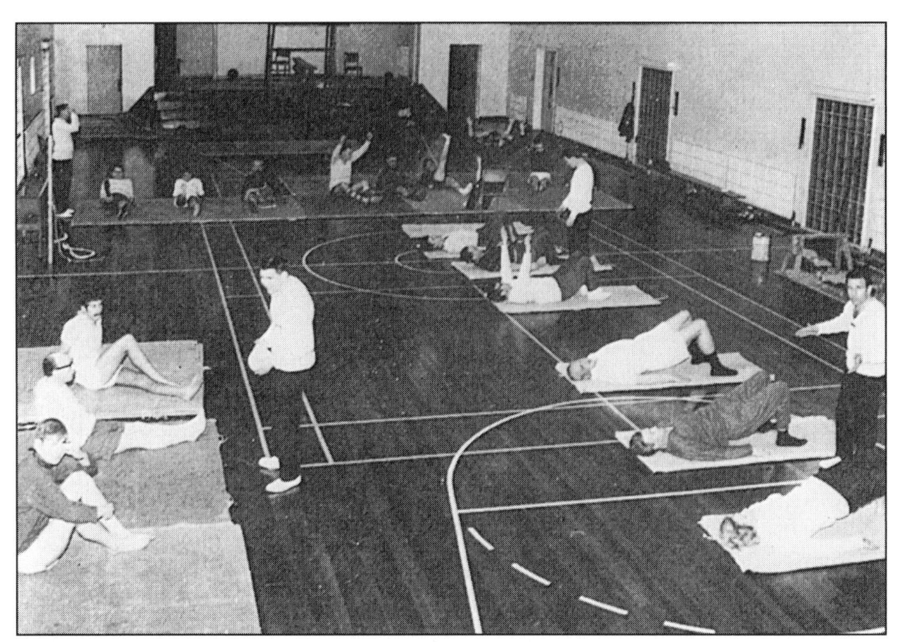

Gymnasium of Headley Court Joint Services Medical Rehabilitation Unit, 1970 (© British Crown copyright/MOD reproduced with permission of the Controller of Her Britannic Majesty's Stationery Office)

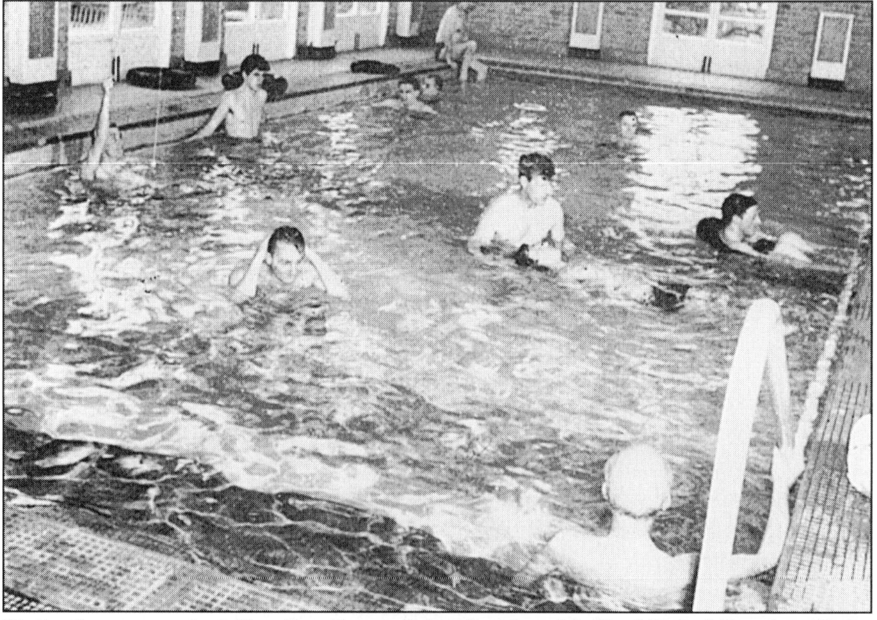

Hydrotherapy pool at Headley Court Joint Services Medical Rehabilitation Unit, 1970 (© British Crown copyright/MOD reproduced with permission of the Controller of Her Britannic Majesty's Stationery Office)

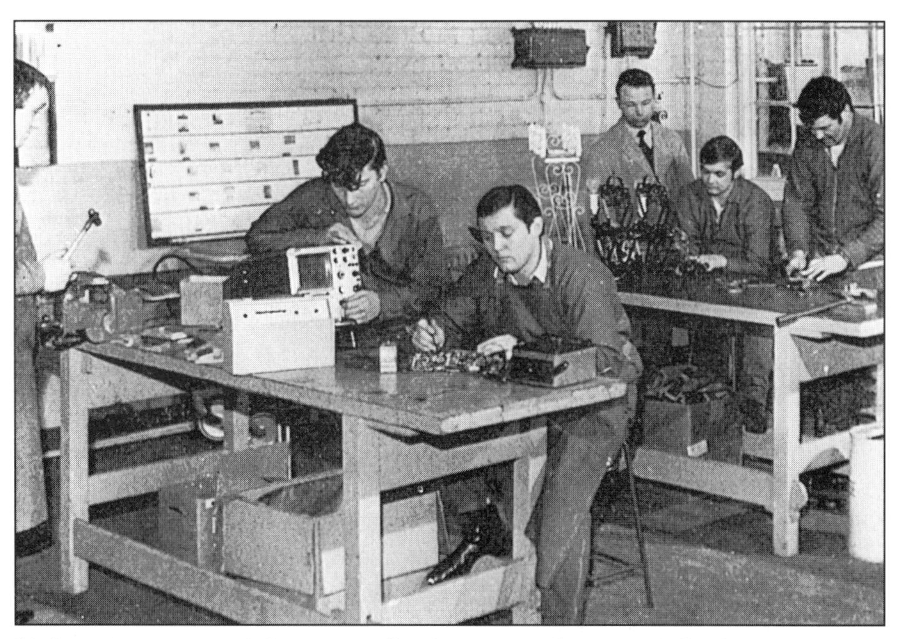

Light engineering workshop at Headley Court Joint Services Medical Rehabilitation Unit, 1970 (© British Crown copyright/MOD reproduced with permission of the Controller of Her Britannic Majesty's Stationery Office)

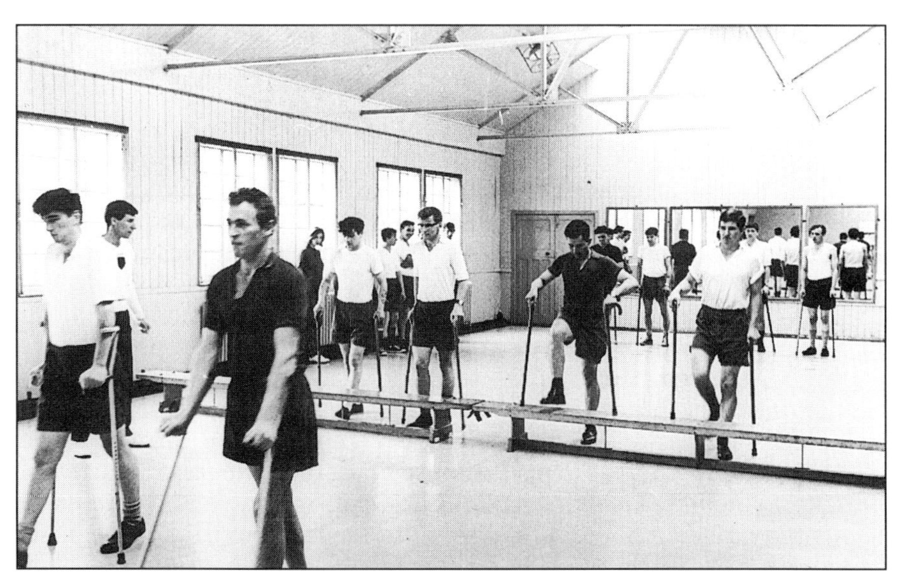

Rehabilitation of amputees, Army Medical Rehabilitation Centre, Chester, 1956 (Wellcome Institute Library, London)

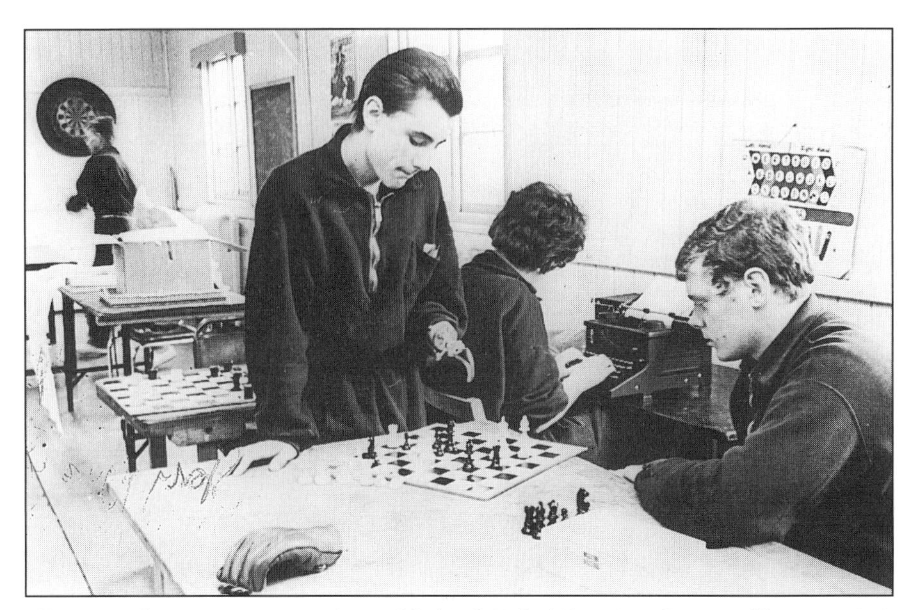

Therapy of arm amputees, Army Medical Rehabilitation Centre, Chester, 1956 (Wellcome Institute Library, London)

and cycle rides. Morale was maintained by dances, games, films and debates in the evening. At a later date units were sited at Hoylake and Cosford, and at orthopaedic hospitals elsewhere. Headley Court and RAF Chessington were the two centres retained when the war ended and RAF Chessington with Headley Court later became the Joint Services Rehabilitation Centre (CB Wynn Parry, 1970) combining with the Army Medical Rehabilitation Centre from Chester.

The Royal Navy

The first naval rehabilitation centre was started at the RN Auxiliary Hospital at Kingslat, Aberdeen by Dr F Godsalve Ward who was much influenced by the work at the Miners Rehabilitation Centre at Benny Hill Hall, Mansfield. This moved to Leweston Manor near Sherbourne in 1943 and Oakley Manor Bromley Kent was opened in 1944. The Centre at Lewston Manor received help from the personnel from Sherbourne School. The accommodation at Oakley Manor was very limited and only about 40 patients could be housed there 'due to lack of washing and lavatory provisions'. In June 1944 the buildings received damage from a 'doodle-bug' and the patients were moved to a ward at the RN Hospital at Chatham and then to St Felix School in Southwold which had been taken over as a rehabilitation centre and remained so till May 1945. There were other smaller RN Auxiliary Hospitals but these were little more than centres of accommodation. At the main centres the type of treatments were clearly influenced by the Army and Air Force experience and were of a similar nature.

Chapter 2

The Foundation and Structure of the British Association of Physical Medicine

The success of these various units in war time suggested that here was an opportunity to establish a specialty of physical medicine and it was Brigadier FD Howitt who persuaded Lord Horder to launch the project, and he also consulted Sir Stanley Davidson. An informal meeting was held at Claridges in October 1942 and a Preliminary Enquiry Committee appointed. The Enquiry Committee consisted of Dr LD Bailey, Dr P Bauwens, Wing-Commander Bromley, Dr Geoffrey Holmes, Lord Horder, Brigadier Howitt, Major JWT Patterson, Dr Donald Stewart and Sir Robert Stanton-Woods. It was as a result of their work that an unofficial meeting was called for 5 May 1943 at the Rooms of the Medical Society of London in Chandos Street. The attendance numbered 60. Lord Horder took the chair at the meeting and a resolution was placed before it: 'That the British Association of Physical Medicine is hereby constituted. The purposes of the Association are to promote a general appreciation of the value of physical medicine in the prevention and relief of human suffering and to implement measures by which practitioners in physical medicine may be encouraged to attain the highest possible standard of efficiency and to use it most effectively for the national well-being.' This resolution went on to define the founder members of the Association and the addition of new members, the summoning of an AGM and the permission for calling any special meeting.

A lengthy discussion followed but eventually it was resolved that 'the British Association of Physical Medicine is hereby constituted'. Problems about membership were referred to the Council (to be elected) for consideration at a later meeting.

The meeting thereupon became the first meeting of the BAPM. The main business of this meeting was consideration of the election of the Council and the powers to be given to it. It was agreed that the Council should consist of twenty members 'with power to act in all matters coming within the objects of the Association'. It was agreed that medico-political questions should not come within the province of the Association. After debate it was agreed that the nucleus of the Council should consist of the nine members of the Enquiry Committee (except Dr Donald Stewart), that eleven additional members should be elected at the next meeting of the Association and that in the meanwhile nominations should be invited for these eleven.

The next meeting took place on 25 May 1943 and, after a ballot, eleven additional members were added to the Council. These were Dr F Bach, Dr W Beaumont, Dr CB Heald, Dr JB Mennell, Dr MB Ray, Dr Kenneth Stone, Major WS Tegner, Dr Dorothy Wood, Dr Hugh Burt, Dr FS Cooksey and Dr EJ Crisp.

At the following meeting of the Council (on 8 July 1943), Lord Horder was elected President of the Association acting as Chairman of the Council for the first year. The Honorary Treasurer—Dr MB Ray; Honorary Medical Secretary—Dr P Bauwens; Honorary General Secretary—Sir Frank Fox were the other officers elected. The subscription for members was fixed at one guinea a year. A vote of thanks to Lord Horder for fostering the foundation of the Association was carried with acclamation. During the first year of the Association three standing sub-committees were set up:

(1) **The Technical and Scientific Committee** (Chairman Dr P Bauwens) undertook the task of assessing equipment used in the diagnosis and treatment of locomotor diseases. It was also responsible for advising research workers in the field and helping to obtain grants.
(2) **The Education and Training Committee** (Chairman Dr Bailey) was responsible for liaising with other training groups, particularly The Chartered Society of Physiotherapists (CSP) and the Post-graduate Courses Control Committee convened by the ERC. However during this period much of the work of this group also involved the provision of courses for the preparation of the Diploma of Physical Medicine and considering the syllabus for this diploma.
(3) **The Policy and Public Relations Committee** (Chairman Dr F Bach) was responsible for obtaining representatives on related committees particularly the CSP and the BMA. It was responsible for liaising with similar bodies in other countries and arranging clinical meetings. It also undertook to explore the possibility of publishing a journal.
(4) **A Finance Sub-committee** was also formed in 1945.

The first AGM was held on 21 June 1944 in Chandos Street when the members met for tea and the President submitted his report (as approved by the Council). Lord Horder could report a fair beginning to the Association. The war had prevented much travel but academic meetings had been planned. The membership now numbered one hundred. Both the medical and lay press had given the Association a warm welcome and a cordial message had been received from Dr Richard Kovacs of the American Congress of Physical Therapy. Dr Richard Kovacs was Clinical Professor and Director of Physical Therapy at the Polyclinic Medical School and Hospital, New York and at the City Hospital, New York. He is well known for his book *Electrotherapy and Light Therapy* which came to five editions in the 1930s. He was a founder member of the Society for Physical Medicine in America in 1932. He died in 1950 and is remembered in the Richard Kovac's Memorial Lecture inaugurated at the RSM in 1961.

The meeting proceeded to the election of Officers and members of Council. A suggestion that the Association should make representation to the Ministry of Health regarding the importance of physical medicine in the Public Health Policy was referred to the Council, and some problems relating to training and gaining experience in physical medicine were discussed and referred to the appropriate subcommittee. The Council elected were:

Dr Francis Bach
Dr P Bauwens
Dr LD Bailey, CB MC
Dr W Beaumont
Group Captain JF Bromley
Dr Hugh Burt
Dr FS Cooksey, OBE
Dr EJ Crisp
Dr WSC Copeman, OBE
Dr J Cowan
Major G Kersley
Lord Horder, GCVO
Brigadier FD Howitt, CVO
Dr James Mennell
Col JWT Patterson
Dr MB Ray, DSO OBE
Sir Merton Smart, RCVO DSO RNVR
Dr Kenneth Stone
Dr WS Tegner
Sir Robert Stanton-Woods

and the Officers were:

President Lord Horder, GCVO
Hon Treasurer Dr MB Ray
Hon Medical Secretary Dr P Bauwens
Hon General Secretary Sir Frank Fox

This council was re-elected at the second AGM held at 11 Chandos Street on 26 June 1945 when the members met for tea. Three scientific meetings were held during 1945: (1) 'The Management of Infantile Paralysis' by the Kenny Method at 1 Wimpole Street, by courtesy of the RSM; (2) 'Sleep Posture—its Implications' by Dr James McDonnell and (3) 'Physical Methods in the Treatment of So-called Psycho-somatic Disease' by Dr Geoffrey Evans.

Further meetings were arranged to take place at Stoke Mandeville Hospital and the Rehabilitation Unit at Roffey Park was visited in the same year. The third AGM on 15 May 1946 was held at the Royal College of Surgeons, Lincoln's Inn Fields, London WC2 when the secretariat moved there from Chandos Street.

In the first years of the Association it is clear that a good deal of discussion took place on the scope of physical medicine and the exact function of the specialist in physical medicine, but it was not until 1946 that the Council made any firm statement of their views. During this period the opinion seemed to have been that 'physical medicine is that branch of medical art which employs physical agents in diagnosis and treatment of disease'. (This view seems very restrictive but in war time rehabilitation was clearly the main priority.)

Autographed menu of dinner after the council meeting of the British Association of Physical Medicine, June 1945, at LeCoq d'or

Presidents and Presidential Badge

In 1954 Dr FD Howitt died. He can with justice be called the 'Father of Physical Medicine'. Although never President of BAPM, it was he who saw 'the need to combine a clinical approach to locomotor disorders with a concern for its physical treatment and for those who carried out the treatment.' He saw that 'treatment was not complete without the rehabilitation and resettlement of the patient.' He had a dynamic personality and succeeded in inspiring those around him to achieve this end. Not only was he one of the founders of the Heberden Society and its first President but also the initiator of the war-time rehabilitation service in the Army. His name has been remembered in the Howitt Club.

He qualified at Guy's Hospital in 1923 and became Chief Assistant to the Skin Department where he became expert in the application of ultra-violet light in the treatment of disease. This lead to his interest in physical treatments and later he was appointed Assistant Honorary Physician to the Royal Free Hospital and Honorary Physician to the Prince of Wales Hospital, Tottenham. In 1929 he was one of the physicians who treated King George V (with ultra violet light). For which he was made CVO.

Lord Horder died in 1955 and many tributes have been paid to the achievements of this remarkable man. It has been said that he was the greatest British clinician of his time. He had been President of the BAPM since its inception in 1943. The obituary in the *Annals*

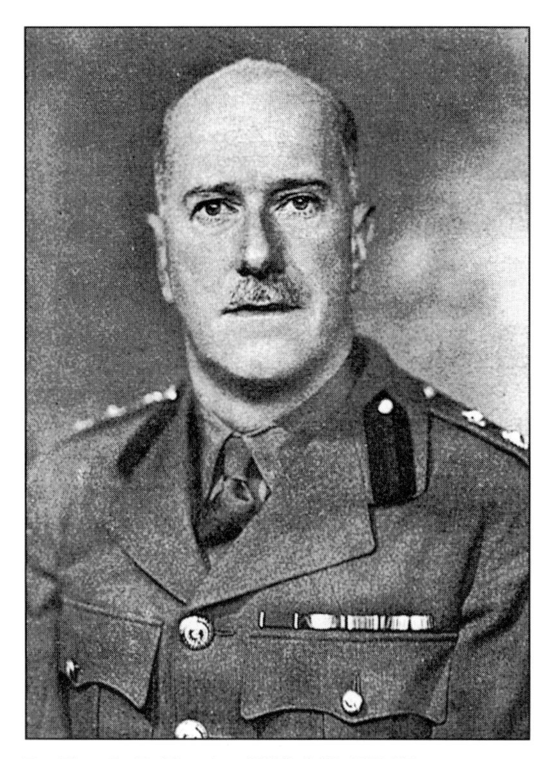

Dr Frank D Howitt CVO MD FRCP

of Physical Medicine spoke of his broad and humanistic approach and the extreme good fortune of the BAPM to have him as its first President. His many achievements have been fully recorded elsewhere. In the rheumatology field he had been chairman of the ERC from its foundation in 1936 till 1953, President of the Heberden Society (1953) and Orator in 1952. As Lord Horder had been President of BAPM for 12 years it was necessary to decide how his successor would be appointed. Eventually it was decided that this should be done by a vote of the full members at the AGM. The method adopted involved each member voting (by ballot paper) for his first choice for President. If one member obtained 50% of the votes he was elected President. If no member achieved this a second ballot was held between the two nominees with the highest number of votes (this is the method used to elect the Pope). The term of office should be 3 years although later in 1974 this was reduced to 2 years. Dr Phillipe Bauwens was elected in this way to serve as President from 1956–1959. A very unforeseen event occurred in 1978 when on the second vote there was a dead heat (between Professor V Wright and Dr BE Mace). A third vote was therefore carried out and this time Professor Wright was elected. Justice however was served as Dr BE Mace became President 2 years later. Soon after the death

Consideration was also given to the recognition of hospitals which would be suitable for training for the diploma. The list was modified from time to time. In 1958 the Association felt that much of the theoretical physics in Part I of the examination was 'irrelevant in the present day practice of the specialty'. They therefore suggested a modification of Part I so that only a general knowledge of physics was required, but with special references to the apparatus and accessories in general use—the number of these should be limited to those with known specific values. It was felt that the diploma laid too much emphasis on therapeutics, whereas more stress should be put on the diagnosis and general treatment of medical disorders of the locomotor system. The criteria for recognition of hospitals for training for the D Phys Med were also discussed. The joint board accepted most of these suggestions.

Annual General Meeting and Scientific Meeting

After the war, the annual business meeting was joined to a scientific meeting. At first the business meeting continued at the Royal College of Surgeons, Lincoln's Inn Fields and the Scientific meeting at one of the London Teaching Hospitals but in 1953, the two meetings were combined at a hospital (University College Hospital). The scientific meeting has taken various forms—in the early years usually there was a discussion session, a clinical demonstration, short papers and perhaps a visit to a rehabilitation centre or a hospital near London. The discussion session might be on a clinical subject—manipulation was the subject in 1952, degenerative joint disease in 1956 and training for physical medicine was discussed in 1953. Visits were paid to the Royal National Orthopaedic Hospital in 1952 and again in 1961; Headley Court RAF Rehabilitation Centre was visited in 1953 and Queen Hospital Roehampton in 1955. The venue for the meeting in 1962 was at the RAMC hospital at Millbank. However, the first provincial meeting on a date different from the AGM was in 1955 at Cambridge, although a joint meeting with the Belgian Society of Physical Medicine and Rehabilitation had been held in Ostend in 1954—the first overseas meeting of the Association. Provisional meetings have continued since and were later combined with the Physical Medicine Section of the Royal Society of Medicine and in 1977 a joint meeting with the Heberden Society was held in Bristol.

The format of the Scientific session of the AGM has varied from time to time. On occasions, there have been guest lecturers; Sir Keith Joseph (the Secretary of State for Social Services) addressed the Association in 1973 on 'The Strategy for the Development of the Medical Rehabilitation Services'.

In more recent years, with the increased size of the Association, simultaneous discussion groups or colloquia were inaugurated. These were first tried out in 1969 and as they proved successful, have continued since. Poster sessions have also been introduced but the most important ingredient perhaps has continued to be the original short papers.

In 1964, it was decided to award a prize of £10 for the best short paper read at the Annual Meeting by a member below the grade of consultant. The paper had to reach a reasonable standard. This prize has continued and in 1974, the Education, Training and Accreditation Committee drew attention to the importance of the prize. It was further stipulated that the paper should report the major part of the work done by the trainee and the author should also demonstrate his/her ability to cope with any questions.

In addition to this prize, in 1980 two new prizes were initiated for essays; one associated with the name of the late Michael Mason in a rheumatological subject and the other associated with the name of the late Philip Nichols on a rehabilitation subject. The essays should be on new work and should be restricted to Associate, Overseas and Full Members of the Association. The value of each prize was to be £100 and awarded on an alternate year basis. The essays were submitted by November 1981, the date for the Philip Nichol Prize was later extended to 31st January 1983.

Annual Dinner

When formal annual dinners were started, they were at first held at the Royal College of Surgeons but this pattern was broken in 1954 when the dinner was moved to Grosvenor House Hotel on one occasion and in 1958 the venue was changed to the Royal College of Physicians which became a fairly usual place after this. Nevertheless, other successful dinners were held at the Society of Apothecaries (1960, 1961 and 1964), Stationers Hall (1959), the Livery Hall of the Guildhall (1963) and the Zoological Gardens (1962 and 1980). Annual Dinners were also held at St Bartholomew's Hospital in 1976 and St Thomas' Hospital in 1982. It was decided largely on the grounds of increasing expense to alternate the dinner with a more informal event.

The invited guests represented a wide range of the medical establishment; often one of the Presidents of the Royal Colleges would be present, or the Chief Medical Officer to the DHSS and representatives of the paramedical professions and the medical journals. Three Ministers have been the principle guests—The Rt Hon Iain Macleod MP Minister of Health (1954), the Rt Hon Derek Walker-Smith QCMP (1960) the Minister of Health, and Sir Keith Joseph (1973) the Secretary of State for Social Services. Dr Gerard Vaughan, the Minister of State, attended the dinner in 1980.

At the AGM there was usually a President's (later a Council's) sherry party for members of the Council and new members of the Association. At the Provincial Meeting, there were usually visits to local places of interest for wives and others with a dinner as part of the social programme.

Chapter 3

Impact of The National Health Service

In 1946, with the approach of the National Health Service (NHS), BAPM was asked (in conjunction with the Physical Medicine Group of the BMA) to make recommendations on the organisation of physical medicine in the new service. In fact a memorandum had been prepared by the Heads of the Physical Medicine Departments of the London Teaching Hospitals and as there was some urgency, this memorandum was adopted by the Council and forwarded to the Minister of Health. It is worth noticing the main recommendations, as these represent the views of the Council at this time:

'Physical medicine is not synonymous with although inclusive of physiotherapy. The former represents the work of the medical practitioners specialising in:

(a) maintenance of health through physical education;
(b) restoration of health through rehabilitation;
(c) conservation of function in chronic and degenerative conditions for as long as possible;
(d) supervision co-ordination of physiotherapy, remedial gymnastics, occupational therapy and associated social services;
(e) medical education and training of ancillary personnel.'

The memorandum goes on to stress the need for the education of undergraduates, and postgraduates. Specialists in physical medicine would need special training, and the D Phys Med should be regarded as the minimum specialist qualification. A higher qualification in medicine was desirable for senior appointments. The Association visualised the setting up of physical medicine departments with (at least in teaching hospitals) a director who would be a full member of the hospital staff. The department would provide full rehabilitation services for in-patients and out-patients by means of physiotherapy, remedial gymnastics, occupational therapy and social services and be in close co-operation with disablement resettlement officers of the Ministry of Labour. The aim was to translate the services which had been available during the war to the use of the civilian population. In district hospitals the department might be more limited—with a visiting specialist in physical medicine. There should be in addition separate Rehabilitation Centres—some generalised and some specialised for specific industries or special disabilities. It was proposed that there should be physical development centres, similar to those which had been developed in the Army, for the correction of physical defects. In addition to these, the specialist in physical medicine would be responsible for the long-term management of rheumatism and allied conditions and therefore would be concerned with the 'investigation, diagnosis, special treatment and research', in these conditions. The specialist would be available for domiciliary consultation and, if indicated, for domiciliary physiotherapy and evening treatment clinics.

Although the care of the rheumatic diseases was specifically mentioned, to some it seemed that physical medicine was an entirely therapeutic specialty concerned more with rehabilitation than with the diagnosis of and research into the rheumatic diseases. Furthermore the criteria for consultant status seemed unsatisfactory in not demanding the MRCP as a basic qualification. Indeed in his presidential address in 1946 Lord Horder admitted that BAPM had been slow in carrying out 'business of an academic and clinical nature'. He believed however that BAPM had achieved its main aim. This was to integrate the three branches of physical medicine namely: (1) clinical; (2) physical development; and (3) use and application of physio-therapeutic methods. He did not think it had been easy to incorporate the various small groups working in these fields, but he pleaded for all concerned to pull together to prevent the disintegration of the whole structure. In his autobiography, he said, 'to suggest that there is room for any conflict between those whose main interest in the rheumatic diseases lies in causation and natural history and those who approach the same problem from a therapeutic angle of physical medicine, indicates lack of clear thinking. The two spheres overlap as evidenced by the fact that the personnel of the ERC founded in 1936 and the BAPM have many names in common'. Nevertheless in this period and in spite of Dr Howitt's plea for unity, there were several resignations from BAPM by physicians who considered that rheumatology should be regarded as a specialist subject in its own right and a branch of general medicine rather than linked to physical therapy and rehabilitation. Indeed one view expressed was that physical medicine would develop in the direction of rehabilitation. At a later date (1962) the Joint Working Party in the Medical Staffing Structure in the Hospital Service (The Porritt Committee) sought to promote this view, which will be discussed later (see pages 50-52).

In 1950 the Council undertook a review of the establishment of physical medicine consultants and junior staff and the number of posts which were filled. Of particular concern to the Council was the shortage of physical medicine facilities in the provinces. The problems arose that although there was an increase in the volume of work, there was a shortage of staff and accommodation and sometimes lack of recognition of the specialty. The Council after discussion felt that extra medical assistance could only be achieved by employing senior hospital medical officers (SHMO)—a sub-consultant grade introduced after World War II—and the use of clinical assistants. The number of registrars was generally being reduced at the time and it was felt that it would be impossible to get permission to employ more. Those working in the provinces were encouraged to take an active part in hospital medical committees. All departments should be 'open'. At this time some physical medicine departments only took referrals from other departments inside the hospital—the 'closed departments'. The BAPM consistently campaigned against this, believing that referrals should be from the GP or fellow consultant to the physical medicine consultant. Not only did the closed department make the physical medicine specialist in effect a superintendent physiotherapist but it also made the physiotherapist a mere technician.

In 1951 the Council reconsidered the qualifications requirement for a consultant in physical medicine. They now considered that: (1) the MRCP was essential for consultant status except in exceptional circumstances; (2) the D Phys Med and much experience in physical medicine were also essential; and (3) the D Phy Med alone was not regarded as adequate for consultant status but a clause was added, after considerable discussion, to the effect that in exceptional circumstances the D Phys Med, with original work and exceptional experience, might be thought as adequate for an interim period. It was felt that there should be some concessions in the period after the war, when there were some senior doctors who had considerable experience in the Services but who had no higher qualifications. Furthermore, some registrars felt that they had been encouraged to spend some years training for the D Phys Med which now appeared to be wasted. At the same time it had to be admitted that there was a shortage of fully trained candidates for the posts which were available and the alternative was to leave the posts unfilled and in the climate of opinion after the war there was certainly a demand for doctors with experience in rehabilitation. However, the acceptance of this situation must be regarded as a factor which had led to the division within the specialty.

It was not until 1955 that the Council, in conjunction with the BMA group, produced another memorandum on the 'Training for the Specialty and Criteria for Consultant Status'. This arose in the evidence submitted to the Willink Committee which had been set up in that year to estimate 'the number of medical practitioners likely to be engaged in all branches of the profession in the future and consequently the intake of medical students required'. The memorandum laid increased emphasis on the clinical side of the specialty—the diagnosis and treatment of the chronic rheumatic diseases and the need for a higher qualification in general medicine. The criteria for consultant status laid down in this document required: (1) qualification for 7 years, 3 years of which should have been spent full time in a department of physical medicine; (2) fellowship or membership of the RCP ; and (3) the D Phys Med was also regarded as essential. The document stated that the interim period and exceptional circumstances no longer existed and that there were now enough fully qualified applicants available. To support this claim it was noted that in the two previous years, of the ten consultant posts, five appointees had the MRCP and the D Phys Med qualifications, three had the MRCP alone and two had the D Phys Med alone. The memorandum went on to encourage the original interests of the specialty in electrodiagnosis, physiotherapeutic methods and rehabilitation.

Developments in Rheumatology

Meanwhile, largely as a result of the introduction of cortisone by Hench *et al.* in 1949, interest in the rheumatic diseases was increasing and efforts were being made to establish rheumatology as a specialty in its own right. Philip S Hench (1896-1965) was Professor at the Mayo Clinic and with his associates, Edward Kendall and Professor Reichstein, received the Nobel Prize for Physiology and Medicine in 1956 for his work on cortisone.

The RCP appointed a Committee for the Chronic Rheumatic Diseases which produced reports in 1951 and 1961. The committee of 1951 (Chairman Lord Brain) recommended 'the establishment of special centres for the treatment of the rheumatic diseases with special training for specialists. These could form a special interest in general medicine or could be combined with physical medicine or orthopaedics. The MRCP or equivalent degree would be necessary for consultants'. Encouraged by this in 1953 a deputation was organised by the ERC for a meeting with the Minister of Health (The Rt Hon Iain MacLeod MP). The deputation was composed of Lord Horder, Professor RE Tunbridge, Dr WSC Copeman, Professor EGL Bywaters and Dr GD Kersley who met the Minister and Sir John Charles (the Chief Medical Officer). A memorandum was produced for the meeting, the aim of which was to establish a specialty of rheumatology with specialists and registrars. The deputation considered that rheumatology as a study was not synonymous with physical medicine. They considered that physical medicine covered a wider field than rheumatology and should also be recognised as a specialty. Dr Kersley records that at the meeting the Minister 'readily agreed but his satellites replied that we already had them (consultants), but that they were called physical medicine specialists'. The official reply given by the Minister however stated that recognition of a specialty depended on professional bodies and not on ministerial decrees. At the same time it was agreed to keep the matter under review. In the next year (1954) a further letter was written to the Minister requesting the appointment of senior registrars in rheumatology, the suggestion made by the Ministry that joint appointments between medicine and rheumatology was not discounted, but it was felt that at registrar level this would not produce consultants of sufficient experience in rheumatology. The letter continued that there was a danger that 'if rheumatology is not recognised, public opinion will consider that men trained in physical medicine are automatically specialists in rheumatology and the ERC consider that this would be undesirable'. In November 1954 there was another meeting between a deputation (Professor RE Tunbridge and Dr WSC Copeman) and Sir John Charles, Mr Pater and the Minister. Arising out of this meeting it was agreed that in the new ministerial circular regarding senior registrar appointments, rheumatology would be mentioned as one of the subjects that senior registrars could study during the course of their training. This commitment was accepted by the executive committee of the ERC.

At a later date, the report of the 1961 Committee of the RCP (Chairman Sir Robert Platt) recommended that '(1) a number of physicians should devote the whole of their time in this field (rheumatology); (2) special centres should be established, at least one in each region; (3) in view of recent advances it was desirable to make a number of consultant clinical appointments in rheumatology; their training would initially be devoted mainly to general medicine and later to specialist training; and (4) in every hospital group there should be a general physician who should devote himself in part to the rheumatic diseases, in some hospitals this might be the consultant in physical medicine'.

The Piercy Committee–Rehabilitation

There were also developments taking place in rehabilitation. There had previously been a report by an Interdepartmental Committee of the Ministry of Labour and National Service on the 'Rehabilitation and Resettlement of Disabled Persons' in 1942 (Chairman, G Tomlinson), but in 1953 it seemed opportune for another survey and the Council of the BAPM was asked by the Ministry of Labour and National Service to submit written and oral evidence to the Piercy Committee on the Rehabilitation of the Disabled. A long report was submitted covering a large range of subjects. In essence the report reviewed the need for rehabilitation particularly after the world wars. It drew a distinction between reablement–the restoration of function after sickness or injury–and resettlement–the provision of facilities for disabled people to earn their living.

The report stated that the whole process of rehabilitation was largely a medical responsibility. This process would involve a team approach which might involve a large number of people. The case conference and resettlement clinics would be the best way of bringing these people together. The wide range of patients who might be involved might mean a very varied approach for different patients. The type of person might vary from (1) those whose function could be fully restored to normal; (2) those with permanent stable disabilities; (3) those with fluctuating disability; and (4) those with disabilities likely to deteriorate. These varying disabilities would require very different rehabilitation centres and because of his training the specialist in physical medicine would play a major role in all the provisions. The Industrial Rehabilitation Unit (IRU) should play an important role at the end of the process. Other provisions desirable were sheltered workshops, home work and day centres for the severely disabled. The disablement resettlement officers (DROs) would play a most important role in the final return to work of the disabled. Voluntary bodies would play an important role in specific disabilities. The occupational therapy department in hospital should provide individual help for patients and this should continue into the home and into the place of work. In conclusion the report stressed (1) that rehabilitation was a complex process involving various authorities; and (2) that the medical practitioners held the necessary training to integrate the medical and social factors necessary for this. Oral evidence was given by Dr AC Boyle, Dr FS Cooksey, Group Capt CJS O'Malley CBE and Dr Donald Wilson. The resulting report of the Piercy Committee contained many quotes from the BAPM submission and followed the general lines of this document.

Paramedical Services

The BAPM had always taken a leading role in promoting the interests of the paramedical professions involved in the remedial services, particularly physiotherapists, remedial gymnasts, occupational therapists and social services. In the 1939–1945 war, the Council had strongly supported the efforts to raise the status of physiotherapists in the fighting services by opening the commissioned ranks to selected individuals.

With the advent of the NHS, the BAPM became concerned with the training and supply of physiotherapists when the Chartered Society of Physiotherapy (CSP) proposed a new curriculum in 1948. A sub-committee was set up to meet representatives of the CSP to enquire into the training, qualifications and examination of medical auxiliaries. As a result of these discussions, the CSP made several alterations to its regulations and syllabus for examination. The Association also issued a memorandum rejecting the idea of physiotherapy aids and recommending the provision of additional training to bring these auxiliaries up to the standard of the CSP so that they could become qualified. They recommended that the best way to overcome the shortage of physiotherapists was to train more teachers and open more schools. They considered that physiotherapy departments should be under the direction of a specialist in physical medicine to make the best use of manpower shortage. They favoured the establishment of a national register of physiotherapists and considered that the only satisfactory examination in physiotherapy was that of the CSP. The Association also gave oral evidence to the Ministry of Health in this subject. At another time they gave written evidence on the employment of blind persons in physiotherapy. The Association continued to encourage links between the two disciplines and welcomed the appointment of a representative of the CSP on the Public Relations Sub-committee of the BAPM and in 1954 at the request of the CSP a member of the Council was nominated to sit on the Educational Advisory Board of their society.

The question of statutory registration continued to cause debate with the CSP; in 1957 the President (Dr P Bauwens) exchanged several letters with the Secretary of the CSP (Miss Nielson). There were meetings between the Executive Committee of the BAPM and representatives of the CSP at which this and the ethical rules of CSP were discussed, together with the ever present problem of shortage of staff. The Council gave evidence to the Cope Committee in 1951 and the amended scheme in 1953. The Councils' views on statutory registration at this time in 1958, were expressed in a letter to the secretary of the Joint Consultants Committee of the BMA. Whilst the Council supported the Statutory Registration of Medical Auxiliaries, they were unhappy about the proposed format. It had been proposed that each of the disciplines (there were 7 of these) should have a separate board whilst there would be a single Co-ordinating Council. The main objection of the Council of the BAPM was that there was an absence in the scheme of effective control by medical practitioners of the training and ethical standards of the auxiliaries concerned. The Council also felt that at that time the training and scope of these auxiliaries was circumscribed and technical and they could not properly be called professions. In the event some concessions were gained on the compositions of the registering boards in that the proportion of medical members was increased but it was not agreed that the Co-ordinating Council should have over-riding powers over the various boards although some agreement was reached on the principle of arbitration in the event of deadlock between the Co-ordinating Council and one of the registering boards. The Government Bill on Professions Supplementary to Medicine was eventually passed in 1960 after a long and contentious course.

The Association had always been concerned with rationalising the use of physiotherapy. In the early 1950s there was a general agreement on the need for scientific investigation of physiotherapeutic procedures. The AGM of 1954 was devoted to the scientific approach. At this time it was felt that too many forms of treatment were passive and placebo in nature. It was recognised that physiotherapy was vital in many conditions but departments were often crowded with patients where it was ineffective. This change of approach had resulted to a large extent in the development of a much more active attitude to rehabilitation with remedial progressive exercises and less dependency on various types of electrical machines and massage. On occasions this led to some conflict with the CSP when some of the older methods of treatment were included in the examination and the final examination still seemed to contain too much emphasis on these treatments. The two members of the Association on the examination board of the final CSP examination resigned on one occasion but eventually the CSP changed the format of the examination. In 1965 a Standing Committee was set up to meet the CSP to study, among other things, the syllabus of the final examination of the CSP. This committee later was expanded to include the Schools of Occupational Therapy and Remedial Gymnasts. Later again in 1968 another sub-committee, the Paramedical Professions Committee, met to advise the Council on all matters concerning the Professions Supplementary to Medicine. The Committee at this stage favoured the concept of a physical therapist having a common course in basic sciences with specialisation at a later stage of training. At the time such an idea did not find favour with these professions. A Multicentre Trials Sub-committee was set up in 1961 to test the value of various physical treatments. The value of traction in cervical spondylosis was investigated, and the value of pre- and post-operative physiotherapy was assessed. A multicentred trial of spinal manipulation was also started. During this period the Scientific and Technical Sub-committee arranged for trials on physiotherapeutic apparatus and, appreciating the possible value of ultrasonics in clinical work, recommended that the Medical Research Council should sponsor research in this field. The Sub-committee was also asked by the Ministry of Health for comments on the requirements of muscle stimulating apparatus and detailed recommendations were drawn up. Eventually a testing plant for apparatus was started at St Thomas' Hospital. The findings were to be published and made available to Hospital Supply Officers. Some summaries could be published in the *Annals of Physical Medicine*.

Relationships with the occupational therapy profession seem to have developed more slowly but in 1949 the Council gave a written statement on the supply, training and qualification of occupational therapists in the NHS. Also in the post-war period, with the increasing use of aids for daily living, modification of homes for the disabled, wheelchairs, walking aids and workshops for the disabled, occupational therapy became a very important part of rehabilitation and the care of the disabled.

In 1963 the Association was asked by Lord Geddes, President of the Association of Occupational Therapists, for advice on a new curriculum for training of occupational therapists. A sub-committee was formed to draw up a reply. They suggested a number of amendments to the curriculum. They suggested that with the widening of the field for occupational therapy there was a need for a great reduction in the time spent on learning crafts which were no longer considered essential in treatment and deplored the fact that the majority of occupational therapists at that time were not associated with teaching centres concerned with other aspects of medical training.

Casualty and Accident Services

In 1961 the Association submitted evidence to the Ministry of Health Sub-committee on Casualty and Accident Services. They pointed out that many physiotherapy and occupational therapy departments were still inadequate and that staffing was also often deficient. They recommended that these deficiencies should be corrected in every hospital with a designated accident centre so that patients could be returned to maximum activity with the least possible delay after accidents.

They recommended that more residential rehabilitation centres should be available in rural areas where out-patient rehabilitation was difficult. They believed that the consultants in physical medicine should organise and supervise the various services and co-operate with the various consultants concerned with the management of accidents. Where junior medical officers were responsible for the treatment of 'casual patients', if physical treatment was required this should be supervised by the consultant in physical medicine.

The Porritt Committee–Medical Staffing Structure in the Hospital Service

The Porritt Committee had asked the Association to submit evidence to it on this subject in 1959. The memorandum submitted was the one already submitted to the *Royal Commission on Doctors and Dentists Renumeration in 1957*. This memorandum had set out to define the scope of physical medicine, the work of doctors engaged in physical medicine and the numbers engaged in its practice. The memorandum recommended that:

(1) there should be further increase in the number of consultants in Physical Medicine particularly in the provinces; this was because consultants not only had clinical responsibilities but also were responsible for the staffing and equipment of their departments and the supervision of medical auxiliaries.
(2) The Senior Hospital Medical Officer grade (SHMO) should not carry out unsupervised clinical work, such work should be done by consultants and the SHMO grade should be allowed to lapse;
(3) there was a need to expand the senior registrar grade;
(4) senior registrar and registrar posts would be more appropriate to teaching hospitals;
(5) there was a place for an increase in the number of clinical assistants.

In addition to this memorandum, two members of the Council gave evidence to the Committee on a personal basis (the President, Dr H Burt and Dr RM Mason). In spite of these views, the Porritt Committee report of 1962 recommended that the specialty of rheumatology should be expanded and that physical medicine should change direction towards becoming a therapeutic service with the emphasis on rehabilitation. The Association was profoundly disturbed by the report and the answers to a questionnaire which followed it. It seemed that the future of physical medicine was being decided by bodies who appeared to be unaware of the practice of the specialty at that time, considering it to be entirely devoted to therapy. In a letter to the *British Medical Journal* and the *Lancet*, Dr WS Tegner (the President of the BAPM at that time) rejected the proposal to create a new specialty of rehabilitation by pointing out that rehabilitation should be an integral part of medical care and the responsibility of every clinician and that to divorce rehabilitation from diagnosis and treatment was unacceptable. As already mentioned, the RCP Committee on the Chronic Rheumatic Diseases (1961; Sir Robert Platt, Chairman), whilst advocating the expansion of the specialty of rheumatology, had accepted that the consultant in physical medicine might be appointed for this purpose.

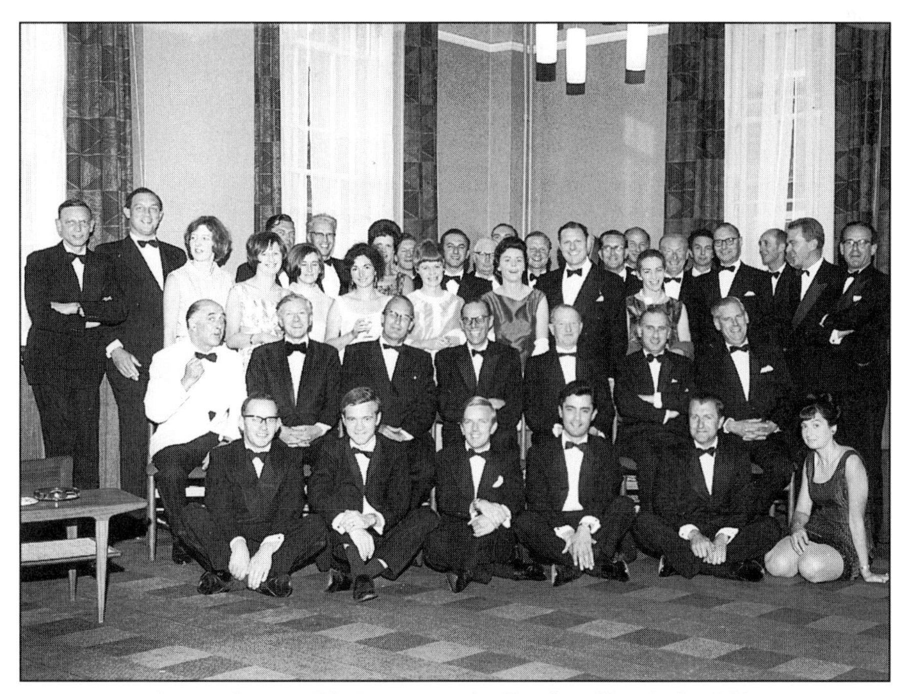

Retirement dinner for Dr WS Tegner at the London Hospital, 1968

seated: RM Mason, CB Wynn-Parry, KN Lloyd, WS Tegner, GO Storey, DL Woolf, Professor HLF Currey

on floor: J Jessop, P Hillenbrand, GRV Hughes, M Seifert, CG Barnes, A Chamberlain

standing front: RA Shaddick, WG Wenley, H Kerr, J Harris, K Norman-Moses, M Brown, M Corbett, J Colston, VL Steinberg, S Hodgson, B Scott, M Zinn, JH Glynn

standing behind: P Nichols, P Knight, M Barnes, B Latham, J Mathews, unknown, M Birkbeck, unknown, N Cardoe, L Bain, unknown, unknown

The Council of the BMA in their annual report of 1963 also rejected that part of the Porritt report which related to this subject (following the advice of the Physical Medicine group of the BMA). The BMA council agreed there was an urgent need to promote rheumatology services but considered that this should not be separate from physical medicine whilst there was also a need for supervision of rehabilitation units. These recommendations however led to further discussions within the BAPM on the relationship between physical medicine and rheumatology and it was suggested that rheumatology should feature in the name of the Association as rheumatology represented the main clinical interest of most of the members. As early as 1961 there had been discussions about this but it was not achieved until 1969.

Dr William Stuart Tegner (1906-1971) qualified at the London Hospital in 1932. He was a founder member of the BAPM and President in 1962. He became Director of the Physical Medicine Department at the London Hospital in 1945. He was on the staff of the Red Cross Clinic at Peto Place and became a member of the staff at the Middlesex Hospital when the clinic was incorporated into that hospital. He retired in 1968 and died in 1971.

Chapter 4

The Journal

The Policy and Public Relations Sub-committee under the Chairmanship of Dr F Bach in 1945 explored the possibility of publishing a new journal for the Association. However, the *British Journal of Physical Medicine and Industrial Hygiene* was already being published by Butterworths and approaches were made to this company to take over the journal as the official organ of the Association. This journal had started life in 1926 as the *British Journal of Actinotherapy* at a time when ultra-light therapy had become fashionable. Eventually in 1946 an agreement was reached; Dr MB Ray was the Editor, to control medical policies while Butterworths would continue to control financial aspects. The name of the journal was to be *The British Journal of Physical Medicine including its Application to Industry.*

The first number was published in February 1947. Dr Burt took over as Editor in 1948 when Dr Ray retired, but in 1950 he reported to the Council that the position, with regard to the journal, was unsatisfactory and the Association withdrew from the arrangement and its name was removed from the cover. *The British Journal of Physical Medicine* finally ceased publication in 1957. It was not until 1952 that the Association published its own journal—*The Annals of Physical Medicine* with Dr Burt as Editor. This was published quarterly with Headley Brothers Ltd as publishers. In the editorial of the first edition, Dr H Burt considered that the scope of the journal should be a wide one. He believed that it should include physical education, rehabilitation and resettlement, as well as the diagnosis and treatment of the disease groups for which physical methods were used. He considered that it should be the place where clinical and technical research should be recorded.

During the first years of the *Annals*, the Editorial Committee was concerned with the lack of suitable material and reports of research, but there was a gradual development in the first five years. Dr AC Boyle took over the editorship in 1955, a new format was introduced and Baillière, Tindall and Cox became the publishers. In 1958 the Editor could announce that the journal had made a small profit.

An Assistant Editor was appointed (Dr DRL Newton) in 1958 in addition to an editorial board and he was followed by Dr S Matingly in 1959. Discussions were held on methods to increase circulation. A special congress number was brought out in 1961 at the time of the International Congress in Washington. The size of the journal was increased to 192 pages, two Assistant Editors were appointed

(Wing Commander Wynn Parry MBE and Dr P Hume Kendall). Mr Papadopulo was appointed Sub-editor. There was however still a shortage of material, particularly original articles.

In 1962 there was a substantial increase in circulation and the demand for back numbers increased. In addition, the amount of material available had improved. The following year Dr Boyle resigned as Editor and Dr P Hume Kendall took over with Dr D Woolf as Assistant Editor.

The success of the journal continued, but the new Editor felt that the Association should spend more on it and have permanent staff. It was proposed to have symposia on drugs and to print the papers which were presented at the AGMs. The summaries were to be collected before the meeting and if the writers wished to publish elsewhere they would be listened to sympathetically.

In 1968 Dr P Hume Kendall died which was a sadly premature loss to the Association, and Dr D Woolf became Editor with Dr J Colston as Assistant Editor. The circulation had now reached 922 and there was plenty of good material; there was a change in format. The name was altered to *Rheumatology and Physical Medicine* in 1969 and with continued progress some papers were being refused. In 1973 the Editor was warmly congratulated in the content and appearance of the revised journal. The name was now *Rheumatology and Rehabilitation* but to avoid raising the subscription, it was reluctantly felt that the accounts of the journal could not be made independent. There was an increase in advertising revenue and

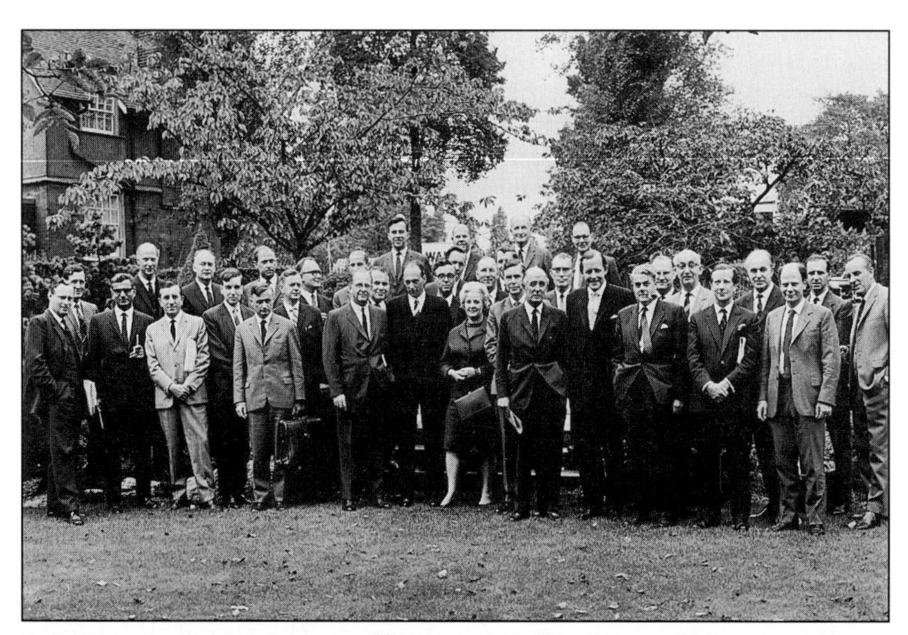

Delegates to a symposium on 'Fenemates', 1966. Among those present were M Simpseen, RM Mason, P Hume-Kendall, AGS Hill and D Doran (in front)

there was more rheumatological than rehabilitation material for publication. Mr Papadopulo retired after 22 years of devoted work to the journal and a presentation was made to him. Mrs Round was appointed as his successor. In 1974 the size of the journal was increased and this resulted in an increase in price. The proposal to publish symposia on drugs was taken up and this increased the revenue which could pay for the rise in price. The symposia were critically discussed before publication to prevent bias. There was an increase in circulation in 1976 to 1290 per issue and the waiting time for publication was 6 months. Dr R Grahame and Dr J Colston were Assistant Editors in 1977 and Dr R Grahame became Associate Editor in 1978 with Dr I Haslock as Assistant Editor. Proposals for a change in name were discussed in 1979; various titles were suggested. Dr Woolf retired as Editor in 1981 and Dr R Grahame took over. The name of *British Journal of Rheumatology* was finally adopted in 1983 and the material for publication was mainly rheumatological. Dr I Haslock, Dr Gumpel and Dr T Gibson were Assistant Editors. There was a slight change of format. The criteria for publication were sharpened and there was an increase in articles from abroad so that the journal could claim to be a leading international journal in clinical rheumatology. In 1982 the publishers Baillière and Tindall were taken over by Columbia Broadcasting System but the Editor reassured the Council that this would do nothing but good for the journal.

Chapter 5

International Congress of Physical Medicine

Discussions had been taking place since 1948 on the possibility of holding an International Congress of Physical Medicine. As an interim arrangement, a committee of the International Federation of Physical Medicine was set up in May 1950 under the Chairmanship of Dr Frank Krusen of America with Dr S Clemmesen of Copenhagen as Vice-chairman with the idea of obtaining international support for this venture. The outcome was that the committee asked the BAPM to be responsible for the organisation of this congress as London was suggested as the most suitable venue and 1952 was suggested as the desirable date.

His Royal Highness the Duke of Gloucester consented to be Patron and Lord Horder, the President of the International Congress. The official opening of the Congress was performed by Marshal of the Royal Air Force The Lord Tedder GCB in the Great Hall, King's

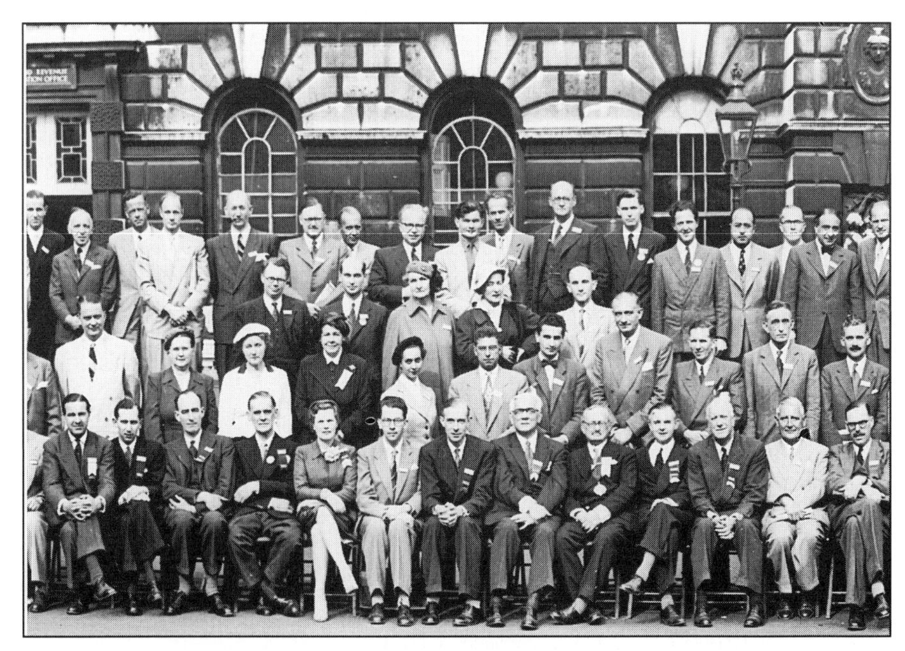

Delegates at the International Congress of Physical Medicine, 1952

front row: AC Boyle, DL Woolf, FS Cooksey, unknown, unknown, unknown, H Burt, F Kreusen, Lord Horder, P Bauwens, F Howitt, unknown, WS Tegner

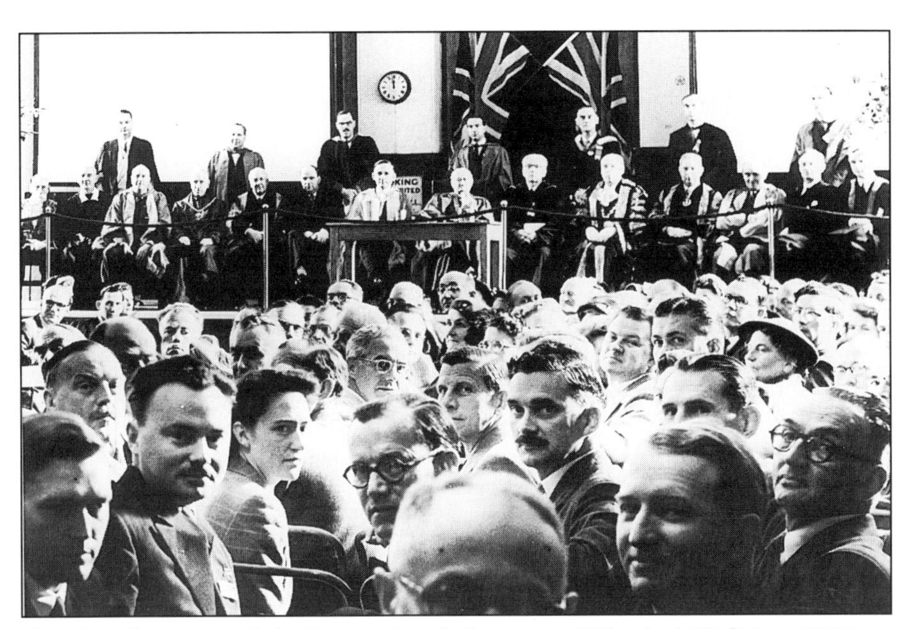

Opening Ceremony of the International Congress of Physical Medicine, 1952

standing back: unknown, F Bach, WS Tegner, AC Boyle, C Shields, H Burt, FS Cooksey
seated: Professor G Bourguignon, unknown, FD Howitt, unknown, Lord Webb-Johnson, Rt Hon Iian Macleod MP, Lord Tedder, Lord Horder, Dr Krusen, unknown, Sir Russell-Brain, unknown, S Clemmenson, P Bauwens
foreground: P Nichols, unknown, EF Mason, N Palmer, GO Storey, unknown

College, Strand, London on Monday 14 July 1952 and the Rt Hon Iain Macleod MP the Minister of Health made a speech of welcome on behalf of HM Government. A ceremonial lamp was lit and the President of the Congress installed. There were representatives of 23 nations present. The scientific programme consisted of various symposia: (1) 'Development in Physical Medicine in the Past Decade'; (2) 'Physical Education';—this included a visit to Aldershot to see physical education in progress; (3) 'Rehabilitation and Resettlement'; (4) 'The Management of Chronic Rheumatic and Other Disorders of the Locomotor System'; and (5) 'Electrodiagnostic Methods'. Exhibitions of aids for the disabled, medical equipment, electronic and electromyographic apparatus was held in adjoining halls.

Films of rehabilitation techniques and physical medicine treatments were shown. The social programme included a reception in Lancaster House, St James on 14 July and a Dinner and Dance at the Dorchester Hotel. There were also visits to Windsor Castle, Hatfield House, Hampton Court and the Royal Naval College.

Press coverage of the congress was extensive. Many press cuttings concentrated on Dr Cooksey's call to get patients back to work after illness, with a reduction of the convalescent period but care for the

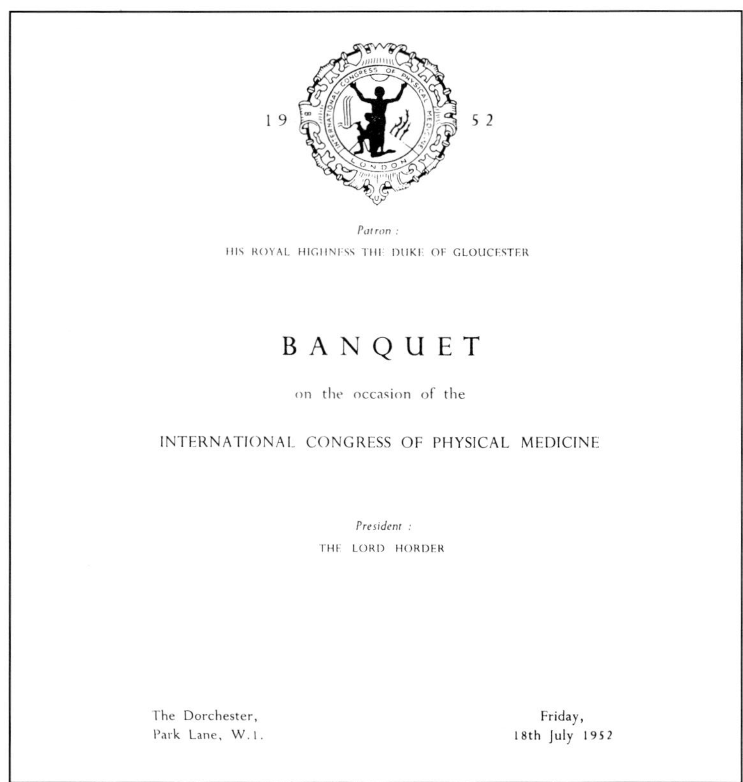

Front of menu for the Banquet at the Dorchester Hotel

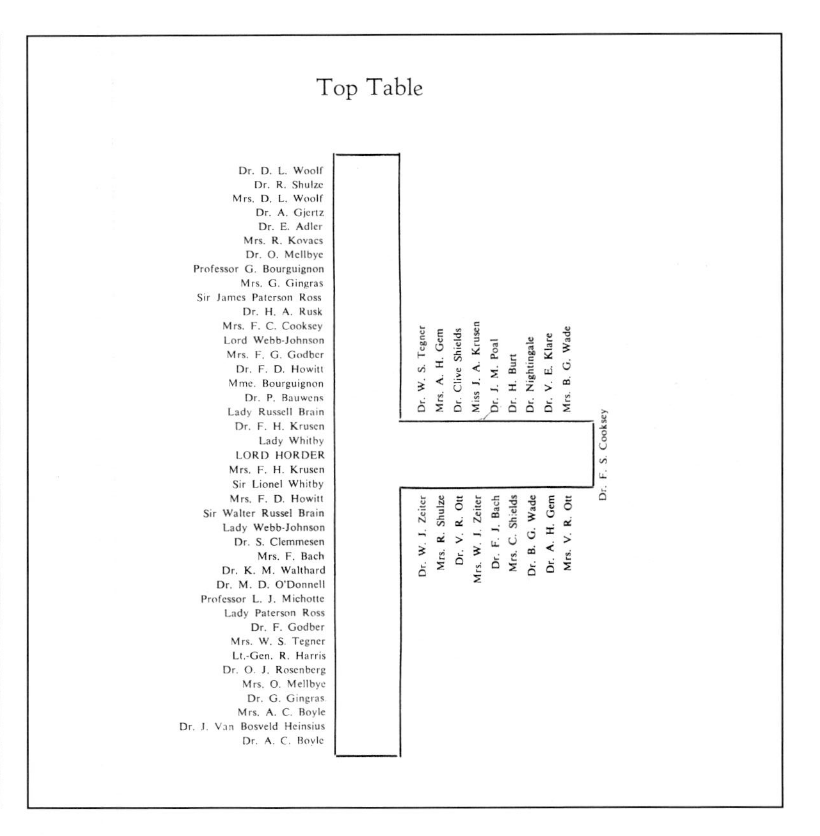

Seating plan for the top table of the Banquet, 18 July 1952

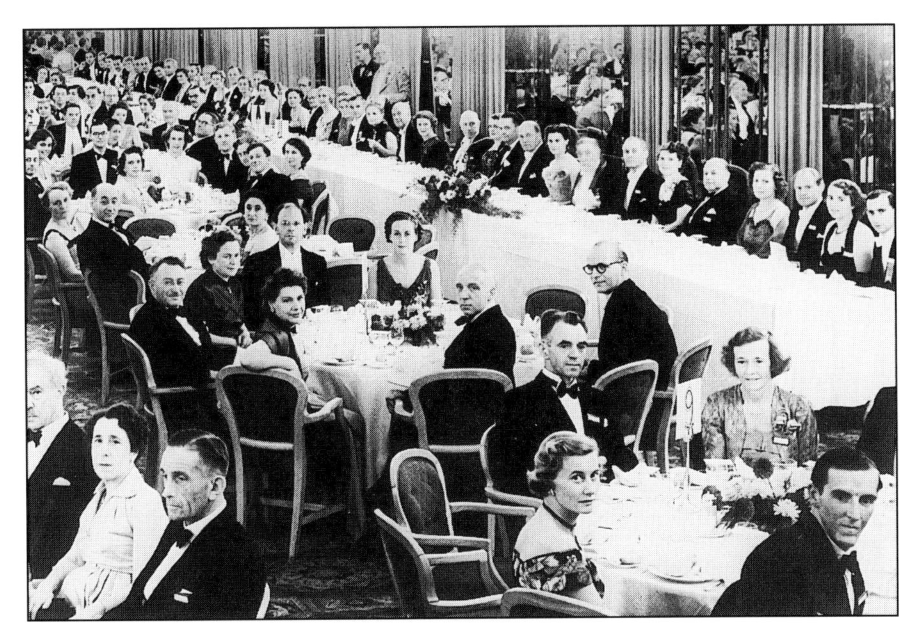

The Banquet, The Dorchester Hotel, 18 July 1952

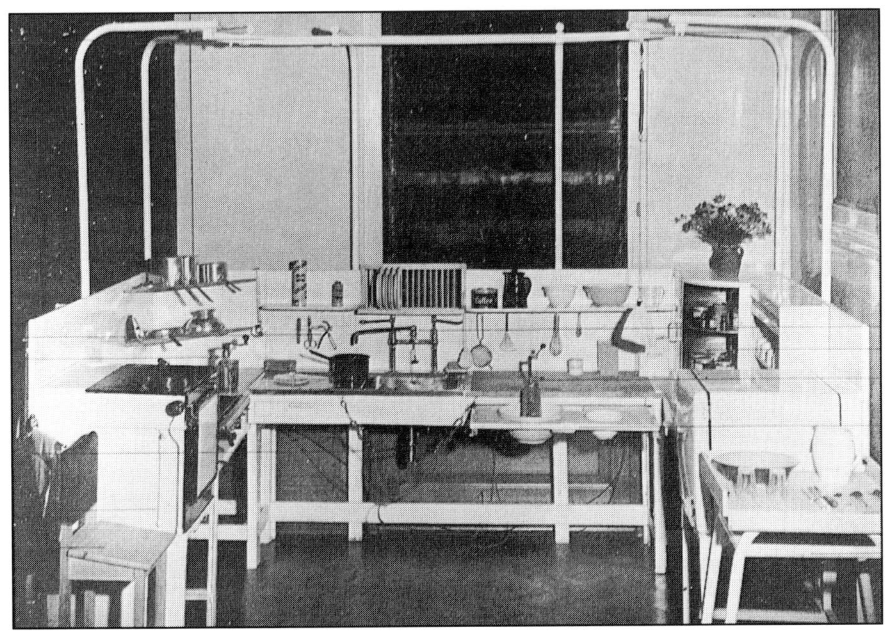

Kitchen unit for disabled housewives, Occupational Therapy Department, King's College Hospital 1952

high chair for arthritis; pilot light for oven; safety belt; tin-opener for use with one hand; easy-grip tongs; sling track; swinging tap with lever handles; rotating shelves; universal grip for grater, mincer, potato peeler and whisk; pull-out board for holding bowl and tin steady; walking trolley (with ramp) elderly and the disabled housewife also attracted attention. A provincial tour was arranged with visits to Birmingham Accident Hospital Rehabilitation Centre, Papworth Village Settlement and Gaston Manor Rehabilitation Centre as well as Stratford-on-Avon, Oxford and Cambridge.

International Federation of Physical Medicine

Before the Congress on Sunday 13 July a meeting of national representatives was held to formally constitute the International Federation of Physical Medicine and adopt the regulations. These set out the object of the Federation which was to advance all aspects of physical medicine which consisted of organising international congresses at regular intervals, improving links between the various countries and exchanging information between Physical Medicine Associations. Dr Frank Krusen was elected the first President.

Subsequent International Congresses of Physical Medicine were held in other countries; the second in Copenhagen in 1956, the third in Washington USA in August 1960; the fourth in Paris in September 1964 and the fifth in Montreal in August 1968. To these congresses the Association sent representatives but in 1968 the President of the Congress expressed concern at the small number of British participants while the Council of the Association expressed disagreement with the way physical medicine was developing in both Canada and the USA. The sixth Congress was in Barcelona, Spain in July 1972 and the seventh in Rio de Janeiro during the summer of 1976, when the name was changed to Physical Medicine and Rehabilitation. It was even suggested in 1975 that the BARR might leave the International Federation but this was not agreed by the Council. Physical medicine in the USA developed in the direction of 'physiatry', a technical and therapeutic discipline treating many conditions.

The Howitt Club

Whilst planning the International Congress, the Executive Committee of the Board of Management were in the habit of dining monthly, after their meetings. It was suggested that these senior members of the specialty of Physical Medicine should get together at regular intervals to formulate future policy. The first meeting for dinner was on 8 December 1953 at the Athenaeum Club. Present were Dr Tegner, Dr Bauwens, Dr Boyle, Dr Burt and Dr Cooksey; Dr Howitt was absent through illness. The rules of the society were drawn up. The name of the society was to be the Howitt Club and there were to be eight members (later this was increased to twelve with three honorary members). Members should retire aged 65 or on retirement from hospital practice. Each member in rotation should entertain the others to dinner and the toast was to be to Dr FD Howitt. After the death of Dr Howitt in 1954 and Lord Horder in 1955, the two names were coupled together and in 1961 the toast was for the late Frank Howitt and the late Tommy Horder; later still other names were added to the toast. New members were elected (only by unanimous vote) and guests attended from time to time, with ladies attending for the first time in 1956. Although the discussions were mainly lighthearted, most of the problems facing the specialty were discussed and it was likely that important decisions on future strategy were taken. Discussions covered a wide range of subjects from the qualification and training needed for physical medicine and the relationship between the BAPM and the CSP, to the importance of the medical disorders of the locomotor system being the central theme of physical medicine. The possibility of a Post-graduate Institute of Physical Medicine was discussed in 1957 (a project which did not come to fruition) as well as the definition of physical medicine. At a later date (1965), the need for a happier relationship with rheumatology was the main concern and in 1961 the rise of 'orthopaedic medicine' was on the agenda. In 1976, Dr PJR Nichols spoke on the future of rehabilitation medicine. In 1969 it was agreed that there should be only one statutory meeting a year and although the club still flourishes, the discussions have become more general and less on policy matters but it has provided a forum for the unofficial exchange of ideas on the developments within the specialty.

Chapter 6

Changing Demands on the Service

Department of Physical Medicine

In 1965 a sub-committee of the BAPM was set up to consider the needs of a Department of Physical Medicine. Their report was completed that year and was forwarded to the BMA. The report was a response to building notes issued by the Ministry of Health. The main points made were:

(1) Although the Ministry of Health building notes had originally been issued as a guide to building a department, they were now being too rigidly adhered to. It was suggested that a consultant in Physical Medicine should be consulted when such plans were being completed.
(2) There was a great need for beds for a department of Physical Medicine; it was suggested that there should be a minimum of ten beds (six female and four male) in major district hospitals.
(3) Suggestions were made on the size of gymnasia and of hydrotherapy pools.
(4) Physiotherapy and occupational therapy should be sited together as one Physical Medicine department. The department should be as close as possible to out-patients and casualty departments.

Physical Medicine and Rheumatology

In 1965 the RCP established a Committee on Physical Medicine. The committee consisted of Sir Max Rosenheim President of the College, Dr K Robson the Registrar with Dr WS Tegner (President), Dr RM Mason and Dr FS Cooksey of the BAPM. The first meeting took place in January 1965. Further meetings took place in July 1966 and October 1967. The College had asked for a definition of Physical Medicine and the definition approved by the College stated that 'Physical medicine is a clinical specialty dealing with the rheumatic and other locomotor (musculo-skeletal) disorders. It is essential, in our opinion, that consultants should continue their role in providing for their colleagues a service of physiotherapy; occupational therapy and remedial gymnastics, and advise when requested on special problems of rehabilitation.' The committee did not think the time was ripe for a change of name.

At the latter meeting it was recommended that the committee should be combined with the rheumatology committee as the Committee for Rheumatology and Physical Medicine and the RCP also recommended that the training programme of rheumatology should be combined with that of physical medicine. The first meeting of the combined committee took place in December 1968 and consisted of Dr FD Hart (Chairman), Dr RM Mason, Dr B Ansell, Dr JT Scott, Dr JH Glyn, Dr AGS Hill as well as Sir Max Rosenheim and Dr K Robson. At a subsequent meeting in January 1970 one of the matters on the agenda was the question whether physical medicine was an obsolete name and whether the committee had responsibility for rehabilitation medicine.

The amalgamation of these committees did not go unchallenged. Some rheumatologists including some junior doctors in training felt that amalgamation with physical medicine would lead to down-grading of the specialty and the loss of potential trainees. They considered that rheumatology should be a branch of internal medicine requiring training in clinical immunology, pharmacology and orthopaedics. They believed that physical medicine had an important but limited role and that there was no justification for the view that the rheumatologist should have charge of the Department of Physiotherapy. The importance of rehabilitation was recognised, as well as the fact that rheumatologists should rehabilitate their own patients. Apart from this there was a need for special centres closely linked with industrial rehabilitation and community social services and they believed that rehabilitation was a viable specialty in its own right. These views were expressed in a letter to the President of the RCP.

However, the combined committee continued for a time and at a later meeting in June 1973 the committee changed its name to Rheumatology and Rehabilitation, and a working party on rehabilitation was appointed to consider particularly the future of the D Phys Med. The working party consisted of Dr RM Mason (Chairman), Dr AC Boyle, Dr PJH Nichols, Dr B Randle and Group Captain Wynn Parry MBE, as well as the President of the Royal College (Dr CA Clarke) and the Registrar (Sir Kenneth Robson). It was this working party which recommended the establishment of the Diploma of Medical Rehabilitation (D Med Rehab) in place of the D Phys Med, which will be considered later (see page 72).

At the 1974 meeting of the Standing Committee, the separation of rheumatology and rehabilitation was discussed and a separate Standing Committee on Rehabilitation was recommended in 1977 (the original committee remained the Rheumatology Committee). The Rehabilitation Committee first met in 1979 as a separate multidisciplinary committee, the BARR being represented by Dr PD Nichols (Chairman), Professor H Glanville, Group Captain CB Wynn Parry and Professor V Wright.

Name of the Association and Accreditation

Informal discussions had been taking place, particularly after the Porritt Committee report, on the name of the Association and in 1969, at the AGM with Dr RM Mason as President, the members voted that in view of the fact that rheumatology represented the major clinical commitment of most members, the name of the Association should be the British Association of Physical Medicine and Rheumatology (BAPM&R) and this name was formally adopted. In August 1969 the journal followed this lead and became *Rheumatology and Physical Medicine.*

Dr Richard Michael Mason qualified from St Bartholomew's Hospital in 1942. After service in the RAF he eventually became Consultant to the Department of Physical Medicine at Chase Farm Hospital. He was appointed Consultant to the Department of Physical Medicine (later Rheumatology) at the London Hospital in 1955. He was Chairman of the ARC and was largely responsible for the opening of the Bone and Joint Research Unit at the London Hospital. He was President of both the Heberden Society and the BARR, as well as the first president of BLAR. He died in June 1977 and is remembered by the Michael Mason prize and medal.

In March 1970, the President (Dr RM Mason) circulated a letter to the members of Council about the proposal of the General Medical Council to initiate specialist registration in view of impending entry into the European Advisory Committees (SACs) and to formulate criteria for specialist registration. The RCP had also called a meeting to discuss the establishing of a Joint Committee on Higher Medical Training (JCHMT); the Heberden Society and the BAPM&R were two of the bodies consulted. The Specialist Advisory Committees (SACs) were to be sub-committees of this committee.

The proposed membership of the SACs were to be: four members nominated by the appropriate specialist association with due regard being paid to the need for representation of specialist academic institutions and of regional physicians. One of the proposed specialties was Rheumatology and Physical Medicine. The Executive Committee expressed the view that the BAPM&R was the appropriate specialist association and the Heberden Society was the specialist academic institution but recognised that this might not be universally accepted and proposed an *ad hoc* meeting with the Heberden Society to discuss this.

The Executive Committee of the Heberden Society suggested the possibility of having two registers: one for Rheumatology and one for Physical (or Rehabilitation) Medicine. Many people would be accredited to both registers. The Executive of the BAPM&R did not consider that Physical (or Rehabilitation) Medicine, as a purely therapeutic specialty, was a viable specialty nor did they think that the Heberden Society was a representative body.

The matter was put to the Council of the BAPM&R who agreed that:

(1) they should press for Rheumatology and Physical Medicine to be recognised as a specialty;
(2) Physical (or Rehabilitation) Medicine as a purely therapeutic specialty was not a viable or acceptable specialty;

(3) the association agreed to participate in a Joint Committee on Higher Training leaving aside the question of designation for the present.

However, at the AGM in March 1971, the President reported that the Executive Council of the Heberden Society was not prepared to participate in a SAC under the title of Rheumatology and Physical Medicine and the Department of Health and Social Security would not accept the separation of the specialties under the titles Physical Medicine and Rheumatology, although they might accept Rheumatology and Rehabilitation. There was a prolonged debate after this with the result that the motion 'This association accepts Rheumatology as the title of the specialty for specialist accreditation' was carried 56 for, 15 against.

The first meeting of the SAC took place in March 1971 under the title of Rheumatology and/or Physical Medicine. Dr A St J Dixon was the first Chairman and the members were Professor JJR Duthie, Dr HLF Currey, Dr AGS Hill, Dr RM Mason (Dr AC Boyle replaced him in April 1971) and Dr DRL Newton (the chairmen to serve for 3 years). The SAC changed its name to Rheumatology in October 1971 and over the years there were frequent changes in membership. As well as being responsible for accreditation of specialists the committee was responsible for vetting training posts and maintaining training standards. The committee drew up the criteria and training required for the specialty of Rheumatology which was later expanded by the BARR as a guide to training. In 1974, a sub-committee on Rehabilitation (SAC) was formed. This included a wide range of specialists (the chairman was Professor C Aitken) and they drew up a training programme for Higher Specialist Training in Medical Rehabilitation which was accepted by the Joint Committee for Higher Medical Training. The programme for accreditation envisaged that there might be various types of doctors seeking experience in rehabilitation. It repeated the belief that all physicians should be responsible for rehabilitating their own patients but that some would take special interest in this aspect of medicine. They would need general professional training similar to that for General (Internal) Medicine but some experience in certain surgical specialties and psychiatry might be included. Experience in cardiology, geriatrics, neurology, neuro-surgery, orthopaedic surgery, paediatrics, respiratory medicine or rheumatology would be particularly relevant. In Higher Professional Training in Rehabilitation the programme required that:

(1) those who intended to take part-time responsibility in rehabilitation medicine were likely to seek accreditation in their own specialty for which they would have to satisfy those requirements. Training would normally extend over two years having clinical duties as well as special interest in rehabilitation.

(2) Those intending to practice exclusively in the specialty of rehabilitation would need: (a) general experience normally extending over 4 years

in approved posts; (b) obligatory experience. The central theme of this training should be the diagnosis and management of physical disability with particular emphasis on the rehabilitation and resettlement of patients with both temporary and long-term handicaps. They must acquire: (i) an accurate knowledge of rehabilitation facilities and services either in hospitals, rehabilitation units or the community; (ii) experience in organisation of rehabilitation services in hospital and the community; (iii) experience in leading a multi-disciplinary team; (iv) experience in research methods; (v) knowledge of conditions in industry; (vi) an understanding of the intellectual and emotional problems of illness and disability as they affect the patient and the family; and (c) recommended experience up to 2 years in a relevant clinical discipline.

In 1980 this Specialist Advisory Committee became a Sub-committee of the SAC of General (Internal) Medicine.

The Tunbridge Committee

A Rehabilitation Sub-committee of the BAPM was set up in 1968. Its primary function was to consider the role of rehabilitation in the District General Hospital. However at the time a Rehabilitation Sub-committee of the Central Health Services Committee (Tunbridge Committee) was seeking evidence on the role of rehabilitation in the NHS. This committee did not seek evidence from the Association as a whole but invited individuals to present personal opinions. Two members of the Association were members of this committee (Dr FS Cooksey and Dr APH Randle). The Council however drew up a memorandum initiated by its Rehabilitation Sub-committee in answer to questions put by the Tunbridge Committee. These answers covered a wide range of subjects and the views of Council at this time on the deficiencies in the service.

The points which this memorandum emphasised were:

(1) Lack of skilled staff. This particularly applied outside the large centres. The shortage was often made worse by misapplication of their skills.
(2) Lack of accommodation. This was a fairly general problem.
(3) Lack of organisation. The need for co-ordination of the various disciplines in a harmonious team.
(4) Lack of medical interest. There was a need for all consultants to be concerned with the rehabilitation of their patients but one consultant should be appointed to organise the rehabilitation service, this might be the consultant in rheumatology and rehabilitation who had special training but rehabilitation alone was not a viable medical specialty in hospital practice. It was necessary for such a consultant to have another clinical interest.

There was a need for the medical staff of all hospitals to reach agreement on the facilities and staff for efficient rehabilitation and see that adequate funding was available.

On the role of various institutions, they considered that:

(1) The remedial treatment service should be concentrated at District General Hospitals as the most efficient way of co-ordinating intensive treatment while skilled staff were in short supply.
(2) Local Authority Services should help the permanently disabled and make available aids for the home and provide occupation centres and social clubs.
(3) General Practitioners (GPs) should be responsible for primary treatment and the long-term care of the permanently disabled. Part-time posts as clinical assistants in departments of physical medicine and rheumatology were particularly suitable for GPs.

The memorandum went on to explore the functions of the various professions involved in rehabilitation: (1) in the hospital service and (2) in the Local Authority service. The sub-committee felt that occupational therapists, physiotherapists and remedial gymnasts were more effective based in hospitals, with perhaps visits to patients' home to advise on adaptations etc. On the question whether one consultant should be in overall charge of the services, the council believed that this should be the aim although the responsibility might be shared. Hostel accommodation might be required in certain circumstances.

With regard to training:

- Medical students should have an attachment to the Department of Physical Medicine and Rheumatology during their period of training and questions on rehabilitation should be included in final examinations.
- Postgraduates should be taught the application of rehabilitation by the clinical specialist to whom they are attached.
- Nurses should have systematic instruction in prevention of stiff joints and postural deformities in bed patients and should encourage patients to help themselves dressing and feeding when they are fit to do so.
- The remedial professions should have a common training in the principle and practices of rehabilitation with specialised training in their specific roles. They should be taught the importance of working together.

When the Tunbridge Committee eventually published its report in 1972 the Association welcomed it. They believed that its adoption would greatly improve the service given to disabled people. The report covered a very wide field and considered in detail all the various groups of disabled people as well as community services, Local Authority Social Services and voluntary organisations which would be involved in their care. In general, the Council observed that the scheme would mean extra consultants and members of the remedial professions. The consultants would need specific extra training. All this would mean extra financial support. They supported the view that the medical and industrial rehabilitation services should be linked and that a Disablement Resettlement Officer (DRO) should work within each major District General Hospital.

However, as the leading article in the *BMJ* stated the main difficulty in the rehabilitation service was that too few doctors were prepared to take an interest in it and train in the subject.

Guide To Training

In 1966 the Association, in collaboration with the Physical Medicine Group of the BMA, published a guide to training in physical medicine. This guide was reprinted in the *Annals of Physical Medicine* of that year. It reiterated many of the principles which had already been stated but later in 1972 a revised version was prepared. This followed and expanded the criteria laid down by the SAC in Rheumatology already mentioned. This version published as a brochure visualised a much wider scope of the specialty embracing a concept rheumatology and physical medicine.

The guide visualised the wide spectrum which the specialty might involve. It stressed the need for a sound grounding in general medicine and the passing of the MRCP examination and suggested that consultants in future might require a greater commitment to general medicine than at that time seemed necessary. However the career prospects in rheumatology and physical medicine seemed best with a commitment to administrative responsibility for paramedical services as well as a clinical service as rheumatologist. There was also a need for consultants working in rheumatology with a limited commitment to general medicine and no responsibility for physical therapy. These posts would particularly involve academic units. At that time the prospects were limited but it was hoped that there would be expansions in posts for highly specialised rheumatologists (at the time there were only four professional units).

Although many rheumatic patients were treated by general physicians there were few posts that could be described as general medicine with an interest in rheumatology. The opportunities for research were emphasised in all branches of the specialty. The Association did not consider that rehabilitation should be a separate specialty in Great Britain. There might be special rehabilitation units for patients with difficult problems but any consultant in charge should train primarily in a clinical specialty.

The guide then went on to consider the training needs. This covered preliminary training where it was felt it was not possible to lay down hard and fast rules. The training needs in rheumatology and physical medicine were outlined along with the associated basic science. It was believed that administration of physiotherapy, occupational therapy and rehabilitation could be learned during the consultants daily work. (Dr AC Boyle and Dr S Matingly contributed a paper on the subject in 1971). Special training would be required by some groups for whom it was not possible to lay down strict guide lines. These groups would include those specialists particularly concerned with: (1) rheumatology alone; (2) physical disabilities other than those due to rheumatic diseases; (3) electrodiagnosis and (4) rehabilitation.

With the establishment of an SAC in Rheumatology and one in Rehabilitation in 1974, two separate training programmes were published in 1975. The programme for rheumatology has been modified over the years and now visualises that after general professional training there are likely to be three types of doctor embarking on higher specialist training:

(1) Those intending to practice exclusively in rheumatology;
(2) Those intending to practice in rheumatology and rehabilitation;
(3) Those intending to practice as general physicians with experience and training in rheumatology.

It will be seen that there has been a shift towards general medicine in the training recommendations but it was always envisaged that these should remain fluid so that they could be adapted to the future needs of the health service.

Chapter 7

The British Association of Rheumatology and Rehabilitation

A further change in the name of the Association took place in 1973 following the AGM of 1972 when the Council was instructed by members to draw up a constitution for a new Association incorporating the words Rheumatology and Rehabilitation. A Working Party consisting of the President (Dr AC Boyle), the Honorary Secretaries (Dr DAH Yates and Dr R Grahame), Dr Bryn Millard and Dr PH Wood accordingly spent a long time drawing up a draft constitution. As a result, an Extraordinary General Meeting was called and then turned into an Open Meeting when the constitution was discussed and accepted (this procedure was advised by the Association's solicitors). The Extraordinary General Meeting was then reopened and the Association of Physical Medicine and Rheumatology was dissolved from 31 December, 1972 and the assets transferred to the British Association of Rheumatology and Rehabilitation (BARR).

The change in name was generally accepted as it was felt that the name Physical Medicine was no longer appropriate in modern medicine, physical treatments had become largely standardised and the term gave the impression that the specialty was mainly therapeutic in its interests. It was also recognised that on the Continent and in America, Physical Medicine was synonymous with Physiotherapy. The journal followed suit in 1973 and became *Rheumatology and Rehabilitation.*

The change in the name of the Association necessitated other changes and the President at the time (Dr AC Boyle) wrote to the Chief Medical Officer saying that the term physical medicine was now obsolete and that in future in job specifications the appointments should be known as Consultant Rheumatologist or Consultant in Rheumatology and Rehabilitation or where appropriate Consultant in Rehabilitation. He stressed however that the policy of the Association remained unchanged and consultants would continue to provide administrative charge of remedial departments if they were the most appropriate person to do so, but recognised that this might not always be so.

Dr Archibald Cabbourn Boyle qualified at St Bartholomew's Hospital in 1941. He was a Command Specialist in Physical Medicine in World War II and Director of the Physical Medicine (Rheumatology) Department at the Middlesex Hospital. He was the second President of the BLAR and occupied all the executive posts in the BAPM (BARR), Secretary (1952-1955), Treasurer (1965), Vice President (1954, 1966, 1974), Editor (1957-1965), President (1972-1974). He was one of the guiding lights of the BAPM and the change of name to BARR. He retired in 1983.

After the inauguration of the BARR there was a rise in the membership. Many of those who hitherto regarded themselves as only rheumatologists seem now to have accepted that the Association could represent the interests of the whole of the specialty and it became clear that eventually there should be one society to represent the specialty. The total membership rose from 375 in 1972 to 410 in 1974 (in 1968 it had been 311). A further change in standing sub-committees took place in 1973. As well as the Editorial Board there was: (1) an Education, Training and Accreditation Committee; (2) an Evaluation and Research Committee; (3) a Hospital and Community Services Committee; and (4) a Finance and Grants Committee. In 1975 a Joint Manpower Committee was formed. The function of this latter committee was to maintain a register of consultant and training posts and details of their nature. Also to promote liaison between the BARR and Medical Advisory Committees in the regions and on the basis of this to provide information and advice to the consultant advisers to the DHSS.

Much of the work of the Association now devolved on the sub-committees and among the subjects considered were:

The Quota Scheme In 1973 the Hospital and Community services committee had considered the Quota Scheme for the employment of disabled people (DP) and their views were accepted by the Association and submitted to the Department of Employment. They recommended that the Quota Scheme should be retained for the present. They felt that the Disabled Persons Register was unsatisfactory, the names of those who sought help from the employment services but who did not wish for their names to be placed on the Statutory Register should be included. There should be positive encouragement to those employers who provided work for the more severely handicapped. There should be improved links between health, welfare and employment services.

Mobility of Disabled Persons At this time recommendations were also made to the Baroness Sharp committee on the mobility of Disabled People and it was noted that a large number of the recommendations had been accepted by that committee.

Research The Evaluation and Research Advisory Committee (ETA), in the period 1970 onwards, supported a number of research projects. These included drug trials of hydrochloroquine and salazopyrine, research into physiotherapeutic methods in a controlled study of isometric mobilising exercises for back pain, transcutaneous nerve stimulation and anti-rheumatic drugs in pregnancy. A workshop in algeodystrophy was started. The dissemination of knowledge of adverse drug reaction and the measurement of joint movement were also subjects which involved their concern.

The Diploma of Medical Rehabilitation

The problem of the D Phys Med also arose at this time. Since the MRCP examination became essential for consultant status and the use of physical methods of treatment had become fairly standardised the incentive to retain the D Phys Med had largely disappeared and it had been noted that the standard of examinees had fallen considerably. At the same time it was felt that some diploma was desirable particularly for overseas graduates who having studied in this country, should be able to achieve some evidence of this on their return to their native lands. Negotiations were therefore started to replace the D Phys Med with a Diploma of Rehabilitation (D Med Rehab). The Working Party of the RCP (see page 63) drew up a list of recommendations for this Diploma. It recommended that:

(1) the examination should be held annually;
(2) a period of two years (approved in advance) was necessary;
(3) the examination should be in two parts: one in general rehabilitation embracing anatomy, physiology, pathology of locomotor disorders and their rehabilitation as well as a knowledge of the organisation of Rehabilitation Departments; the second part would be in a special subject (approved in advance) from a choice of neurology, neurosurgery, paediatrics, geriatrics, sports medicine or rheumatology)—this could involve a presentation of 12 case histories or a dissertation of a special clinical study.

The candidates must have fully registrable qualifications or if temporary must produce evidence of their temporary registration.

A syllabus was drawn up for the guidance of candidates. Dr PJR Nicholls was appointed adviser to the Joint Board on the new Diploma with Dr CB Wynn Parry MBE, as adviser to overseas doctors. The list of hospitals approved for the D Phys Med was allowed to lapse and candidates were to be advised by the postgraduate adviser on suitable units. These recommendations were accepted and the first examination for the D Med Rehab was held in 1976.

Post-graduate Courses

The suggestion for post-graduate courses in Physical Medicine originated in 1952. Initially it was suggested that there should be a weekend course and Saturday morning lectures. These courses continued to be held annually and in 1959 it was agreed that one should involve basic matters and one be an advanced course. A separate committee for organising them was set up but this was later fused with the Training Sub-committee. In that year (1959) an approach was made to the British Postgraduate Medical Federation to seek their help to facilitate training particularly for the D Phys Med. The federation promised help in publicising the activities of the Association and to improve this liaison an educational advisor was appointed. Dr H Burt, the President at the time, was elected to fill this post in the first instance.

In 1961 a course of lectures was started particularly for those taking the D Phys Med lasting a full week and it was agreed that not more than two additional courses of an advanced nature should be held during the year. Dr Burt gave up the post of Medical Adviser in 1963 and a postgraduate advisory committee was formed in his place (Dr S Mattingly, Dr AT Richardson and Wing Commander Wynn Parry MBE, Chairman; Dr D Brewerton became postgraduate adviser in 1970). In addition to these, study courses on rehabilitation were started in 1962 and on electrodiagnosis in 1965 and these have continued on a regular basis since. Various other series of lectures were organised on subjects of current interest, for example proprioceptive neuromuscular facilitation at the Westminster Hospital in 1960 and four lectures were given in a course for GPs organised by the Postgraduate Medical Foundation. These courses were held in London, and the problem of the provinces remained until much later when the provincial centres became more developed. It was also felt that overseas graduates needed special experience in the management of a wide range of disabilities and it was suggested that multidisciplinary training courses should be arranged.

In 1974 because of the multiplicity of courses, it was proposed to form a Joint Standing Advisory Committee on meetings and courses. This would involve the Heberden Society, the RSM Section of Rheumatology and Rehabilitation, the British League against Rheumatism (BLAR) and the British Association of Rheumatology and Rehabilitation (BARR). The Association would be represented by the President and Honorary Secretary. In fact, in 1975 it was proposed to hold basic and advanced courses in rehabilitation, as well as courses in electrodiagnosis, both basic and advanced and there were continuing courses in rheumatology at all levels. A course in spinal manipulation was started at St Thomas' Hospital in the same year. To these were added a 'Paediatric Rheumatology' course in 1978, a 'Soft Tissue and Sports Injury' course in 1977/78, and a further course on 'Clinical Problems Peculiar to Sport' in 1978. Later again, with the widening of the field of interest, there were courses in 'Orthotics and Prosthetics Today' in 1979, 'Rheumatic Problems of the Elderly' in 1980, 'Pathology of Rheumatic Diseases' in 1980 and 'Rehabilitation of the Physically Disabled' in 1980. These courses, initiated by the Education Training and Accreditation Sub-committee were organised by various members of the Association and eventually covered the whole field of the specialty. They have continued since with minor variations.

Financial Matters

In the early years of the Association there were small rises in the annual subscription from 1 guinea a year at the start; in 1954 the subscription was £5.5s 0d for Fellows and £2.12s 0d for Members. (Fellows were consultants and Members were other medical practitioners). The designation of Fellow was later dropped in favour of Member and Associated Member. Trustees were to be elected by the Council. The first two were Dr MB Ray and Dr P Bauwens. The Association was registered as a charity in 1959 when there was enough money for some investments. In 1967 it was decided to set up a separate Research and Education Trust Fund. The aims of the fund were:

(1) to encourage research with grants and fellowships of medical research institutions;
(2) to provide laboratories or equipment for laboratories;
(3) to enable overseas doctors to obtain training in Great Britain or doctors from Great Britain to obtain experience overseas;
(4) to publish the results of research;
(5) to make subscriptions or donations to medical schools or other institutions. The Fund could also benefit from donations and legacies. The fund required separate trustees and the President, Immediate Past President and Honorary Treasurer were elected as trustees in the first instance. Two thousand pounds of invested capital was transferred to the Fund at its formation.

In 1968 there was a rise in the subscription to Members, from 6 guineas to £10. This was mainly because the publishers had increased the price of the journal and the Joint Secretariat was costing more. The subsidy from the Council for the Annual Dinner was ceasing and it was also agreed that in future there should be a registration fee for the AGM (up till that time there had been no such fee).

In 1974 the assets of the Research and Education Fund were transferred to the care of the Official Custodian for Charities and the Trust Fund Trustees were separated from the Association's Trustees. To achieve this, a Finance and Grants Advisory Committee was formed. The whole council would act as Trustees for the Research and Education fund but would be advised by the Finance and Grants Advisor Committee. In the event it seems the trustees of the Association acted in both capacities. The funds of the Association had already been transferred to the Official Custodian in 1973. By now in 1975 the effects of inflation were being more severely felt and although there was both an increase in membership and the various courses were well attended, it became necessary to raise the subscription from £10 to £15 for Members and £5 to £7.50 for Associate Members. At the time, the Treasurer (Dr Rodney Grahame), in his letter to Members, summarised the value of the Association:

(1) The BARR is the representative body for those working/or training in both fields of clinical rheumatology and rehabilitation. Its council and committees keep a constant watch on developments both within the specialty and without.
(2) The Research and Education Trust is available to grant (albeit modest) sums of money to promote research and educational projects.
(3) Through affiliation, membership of the BARR confers membership of the British League Against Rheumatism (and through the BLAR to the European and International Leagues) and of the International Federation of Physical Medicine and Rehabilitation.
(4) The Association operates an advisory service for the benefit of those seeking training in the specialty.
(5) The Association organises two scientific meetings of high calibre each year as well as many courses in various aspects of the specialty.
(6) The Association publishes a first-class journal four times yearly.

The better usage of the Research and Education Trust Fund was again raised in 1980 by the treasurer at that time (Dr JH Cosh). As a result, the Evaluation and Research Advisory Committee felt that although the fund was small (£7384 at the time), there were certain advantages in this—they believed the fund could support projects, reports and reviews and it could assist young rheumatologists with foreign travel. A few grants had already been made to individual research projects being undertaken by members unable to get support elsewhere. It was also used to fund the Association Prize given to the best short paper by a Registrar or Senior Registrar at the AGM and at the same time the Committee proposed that two new prizes should be established; one for an essay on a rheumatological subject associated with the name of the late Michael Mason and the other for an essay on a rehabilitation subject associated with the name of the late Philip Nichols. It was suggested that the entries should be restricted to Associate, Overseas and Full Members of the Association. The value of each prize should be £100. They should be awarded on alternate years. The prizes were to commence in 1982.

In 1981 the Association received £3750 on the winding up of the Charterhouse Rheumatism Clinic in Weymouth Street. A further rise in the subscription to £25 for Members took place in 1982.

Chapter 8

Further Developments

Electrodiagnosis

Further developments were taking place in the field of electrodiagnosis. On the technical side, nerve conduction studies were developing. Motor nerve conduction time had been in use since 1948 by Hodes and sensory nerve conduction had been recorded through the skin in man by Dawson and Scott in 1949. Gilliat and Sears had further developed this technique in 1958 but a simpler and easier method for measuring sensory and motor conduction times using antidromic impulses was developed by Campbell and Styles (reported by Campbell in 1962).

In 1959 an International Conference was held in Pavea with the aim of standardising the various terms used in electrodiagnosis and in 1961 the possibility of forming a British Electromyography (EMG) Society was discussed. A letter was received by the BAPM from Dr JM Walton, the Chairman of the Electroencephalography (EEG) Society, suggesting some link up between the two interests. Dr Bauwens, Dr Richardson and Wing Commander Wynn Parry were appointed as a sub-committee to liaise with the EEG Society. As a result, it was decided to form a forum at which there would be opportunities to present papers and discuss subjects of mutual interest. It was felt there was no need for a separate EMG Society but that meetings should be organised annually with the EEG Society. The meetings should be called Symposium on Applied Neuromuscular Physiology. The first meeting was held at the Royal Free Hospital in November 1962. A further international meeting on EMG was held in Copenhagen in 1963 at which the BAPM representatives took part on the organising committee. In view of this meeting the joint meeting with the EEG Society was cancelled for that year.

In 1964 it was agreed that the Association should pay an annual subscription to the International Federation of EEG and Clinical Neurophysiology on the basis that about half the members of the Association undertook EMG work. However, joint meetings between the two gradually diminished.

An international meeting on EMG was held in Glasgow in July 1967. Courses in electrodiagnosis continued on a regular basis organised by the BARR into the 1980s and in spite of an increase in numbers of neurological electrophysiologists, many members still provide an electrodiagnostic service to their hospitals.

The Remedial Professions

In 1972, partly as a result of the Tunbridge report, the remedial professions (occupational therapists, physiotherapists and remedial gymnasts) expressed disappointment to the Secretary of State (Sir Keith Joseph) at the lack of recognition of the skills and services they had to offer the community. As a result, he set up a working party consisting of representatives of these professions and the DHSS under the chairmanship of Mr EL McMillan. The report published by them in 1973 reviewed the various reasons for their dissatisfaction. It also considered the relationship within the remedial professions and their relationship with the medical, nursing and social work professions and with other staff involved in remedial work. The career structure, training and renumeration of therapists were also reviewed.

Among the recommendations which seemed particularly important to the medical profession were:

(1) that therapists should be given a greater measure of freedom and responsibility. They should co-ordinate, organise and administer their own services;
(2) while doctors should provide a diagnosis and state the aims of treatment (subject to later review), the therapists should determine the nature and duration of treatment;
(3) when working in the community the physician best placed to co-ordinate the therapists' services might be the Community Physician.

In addition, the report recommended that the professions of physiotherapy and remedial gymnastics should amalgamate and that in the long term all three professions should form one comprehensive service. The report also recommended the establishment of therapists at district level with management responsibilities, the expansion of the use of aides and the consideration of the establishment of a degree course for remedial therapists. As a response to the report, the President of the Association (Dr DRL Newton) in July 1974 wrote to the Senior Medical Officer of the DHSS, suggesting that there was a need for overall responsibility for rehabilitation at district level and that District Community Physicians (DCPs) were unlikely to have such experience. He pointed out that with the shortage of therapists there might well be no therapist in some districts experienced enough to act as district therapist, and that in many places co-operation between members of individual professions was sadly lacking. He believed that if there were insufficient consultants to provide overall advice on rehabilitation at district level, a consultant should be appointed at area level with this responsibility.

In spite of this letter, the DHSS issued a Health Circular (HSC(15)101) in December 1974 giving guidance to Health Authorities as an interim measure. This required authorities to designate senior therapists of the three professions who 'with medical advice would advise District Community Physicians on the organisation of their services'. These therapists would be accountable to the District Community Physicians for the organisation of their services. The Community Physician would require medical advice on clinical matters and if this was not available at district level, then it should be provided by a designated consultant at area level. It is worth noting that in the reorganisation of the health service which was taking place at this time the post of community physician had been introduced and there was a good deal of uncertainty about exact responsibilities which should be allocated to it.

This circular caused great disquiet among the members of the Association and in March 1975 the President wrote again to the Chief Medical Officer. While welcoming the proper recognition to be given to the remedial professions and the right to administer their own service, he expressed concern that the only interpretation that could be placed on the circular was that the sole medical responsibility for hospital rehabilitation should be rested in the District Community Physician. He pointed out that rehabilitation in hospital was entirely a clinical matter of consultants working in a team with the remedial professions and that a split structure could only lead to confusion and a deterioration in the service.

Following a reply from the DHSS a meeting took place on October 1975 between some members of the Association and the DHSS. The group representing the BARR consisted of the President (Dr DRL Newton), Dr DN Brewerton, Dr PHN Wood, Dr BEW Mace, Professor HJ Glanville and Dr D Zutshi; Dr P Nichols was present as Consultant Advisor to the DHSS. Dr Gillian Ford, Dr M Prophet and Miss P Witherton represented the DHSS. The members of the BARR were concerned about the apparent change in role which consultants in rheumatology and rehabilitation were being asked to adopt. They were worried about these changes having an adverse effect on junior staff who were uncertain about their future—as there was a lack of expertise in rehabilitation and the vacuum might be filled by doctors without clinical training. It was important that clinical specialists should co-ordinate the rehabilitation services. The conclusion reached at the meeting was that a small working party should be set up to identify these problems and attempt to solve them. It was recognised that other interested parties would have to be consulted and that a decision on the final outline of the service would take some time to negotiate. This working party was eventually established as a multidisciplinary committee with representatives from the remedial professions, the DHSS and community medicine (Dr Mace and Dr G Cochrane represented the BARR). A number of meetings were held over a period of about 2 years or more and during this period the DHSS issued other health circulars. HC(77)33 (1977) contained a statement from the Standing Medical Advisory

Committee to the Government on the relationship between the medical and remedial professions. This made various points, the important ones seem to be that the doctor who referred the patient for therapy was not handing over his overall control of the patient but that in asking for treatment the doctor was asking for help from another trained professional. It followed that the therapist had a duty and a right to decline to perform any therapy which the therapist considered to be actively harmful to the patient and the doctor who was responsible for the patient had the right to instruct the therapist not to carry out certain forms of treatment which he believed harmful. Finally the DHSS issued circular HC(79)19 (1979) which superseded HC(15)101 which was cancelled. The circular gave guidance on the management of the remedial professions. It left unchanged the overall medical responsibility for the organisation of the rehabilitation services. It reiterated the need for the remedial therapists to manage their own affairs and the recommendation for the establishment of 'District Therapists' with the establishment of secretarial support. The clinical responsibilities would remain as outlined in circular HC(77)13. It still recommended that relations with the district management team should be through the District Community Physician. In addition to this it strongly recommended the establishment of 'major users' committees to provide advice to the Management Committee on the rehabilitation services. The Association felt that the new circular was an improvement on the old although some of the definitions remained blurred. The Association also considered that the major users committee should be made mandatory in all districts, which the DHSS was unwilling to do and indeed later experience suggested that there was not a great deal of interest outside the Association for these.

During this time, the President of the BARR had met the President of the Faculty of Community Medicine Dr WG Harding in 1976 and established good relations with the Faculty. The community physicians had stated they had no interest in taking on clinical responsibility for which they had no expertise. The Presidents' letter to the DHSS in 1976 had also been published in *Physiotherapy* which had eased relations with the remedial professions.

Rehabilitation

For several years there had been suggestions that rehabilitation was a separate discipline from rheumatology and could be a specialty in its own right. At first this suggestion had been resisted by the Council of the BAPM (BARR) for the reasons already discussed. However, particularly when amalgamation with the Heberden Society became a possibility, the question became more urgent as it was clear that some members of the Heberden Society were unwilling to become involved in rehabilitation (other than when it involved rheumatic patients) and it became clear that rehabilitation

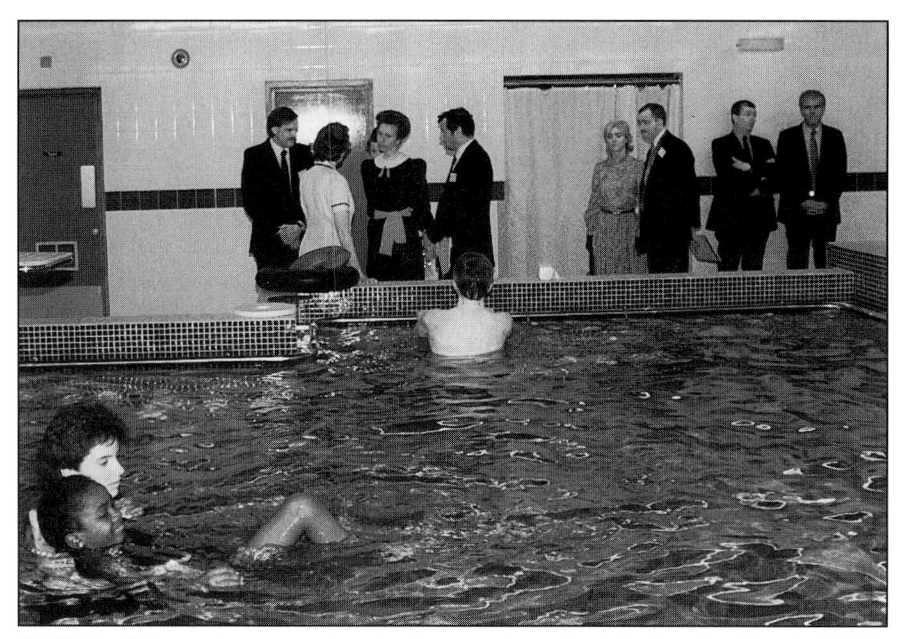

HRH the Princess Anne opening the therapeutic pool at The London Hospital, Mile End, 1987

with her: JD Perry, Miss J Dyer, B Roper

was really a multidisciplinary exercise. The important role of physiotherapy and pool therapy in the treatment of rheumatic patients has of course continued. As has already been stated the Rheumatology and Rehabilitation Committee of the RCP had agreed in 1974 that it would be an advantage if rehabilitation became a specialty in its own right and in 1977 reiterated this view and suggested that there was a place for a consultant in rehabilitation. The separate multidisciplinary Rehabilitation Committee was therefore created (Chairman Dr PJR Nichols) which met for the first time in 1979. The Specialist Advisory Committee in Rehabilitation having been formed in 1974, transferred to General (Internal) Medicine in 1980. These two committees on rehabilitation were to work closely together. The committees assembled detailed evidence on rehabilitation throughout the country to advise any specialty on these facilities. To mark the Year of the Disabled in 1981, the RCP allocated two days of its course on advanced medicine to the consideration of rehabilitation. As well as these developments, the BARR had discussed the Association's responsibility for rehabilitation at its AGM in 1976 and the Hospital and Community Services Committee (Chairman, Dr D Brewerton) had prepared a document which was included in the Association's report to the Royal Commission on the NHS (the Merrison Committee—see page 85) and Dr PJR Nichols published a document *Rehabilitation: Subject*

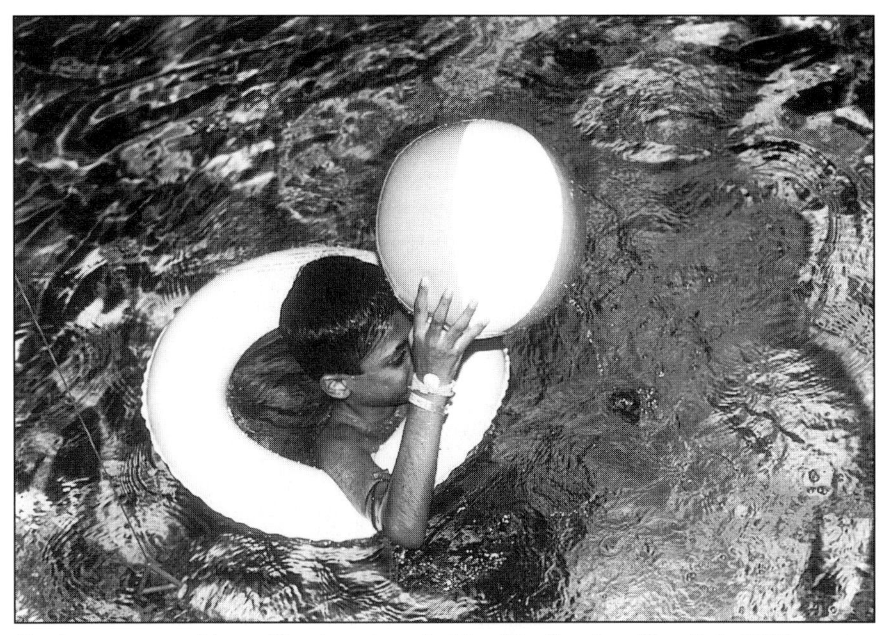

Pool treatment of juvenille chronic arthritis. The London Hospital, 1987

or Specialty. In addition, a questionnaire had been circulated by Dr PHN Wood to members on their responsibility for rehabilitation, and there had been many helpful letters received particularly from junior members. All this evidence supported the view that rehabilitation should be written into the senior registrar accreditation of every specialty and be separated from rheumatology.

Dr A Zinovieff was awarded an OBE for his work in rehabilitation. The establishment of Chairs in Rehabilitation provided another step in the separation of rehabilitation. In 1977 Dr HJ Granville was appointed to the European Chair of Rehabilitation established at the Nuffield Rehabilitation Centre (University of Southampton), in honour of the entry of this country into the European Common Market, and Dr Cairns B Aitken was appointed Professor of Rehabilitation Studies at the University of Edinburgh and more recently, Dr MA Chamberlain (1988) was appointed Professor in Rheumatological Rehabilitation.

In 1981 further discussion on the relationship between rheumatology and rehabilitation took place and Dr Mace (the President) expressed the view that rehabilitation medicine was not benefitting from its association with rheumatology and that the time had come to separate the two subjects. The Council supported this view although it was emphasised that the Association should not abandon rehabilitation medicine until it was fully established. With this in view a standing committee on rehabilitation medicine was set up with Dr G Cochrane as chairman and 14 others representing many

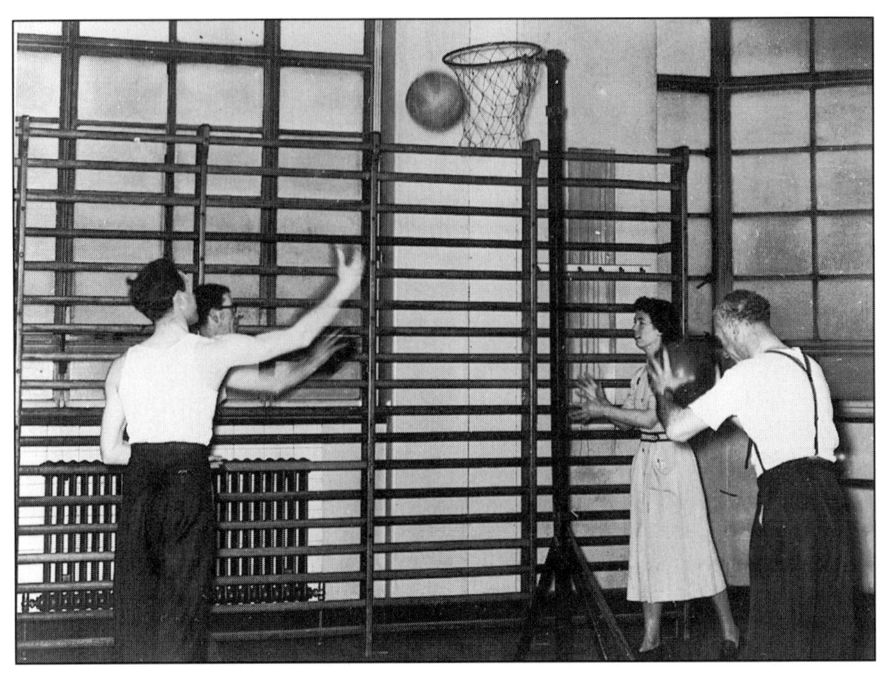

Rehabilitation by games, The London Hospital, 1955

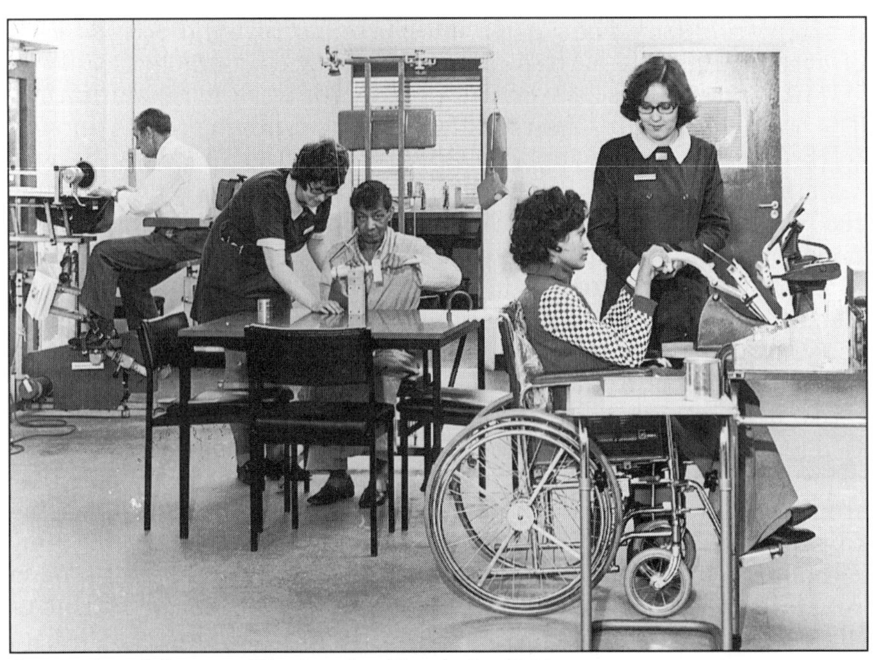

Occupational therapy, The London Hospital, c1980

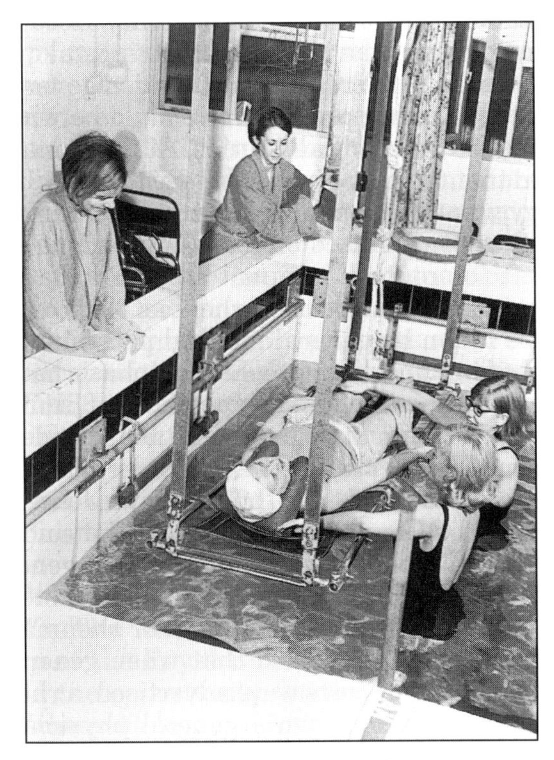

Pool therapy, The London Hospital, 1964

disciplines. The Committee submitted a report on 1 December 1982 reviewing the various agencies and societies which were interested in rehabilitation and recommending the establishment of a medical clinical fellowship to be called the 'Group for the Management of Disability'. The group should be affiliated to the Society for Research in Rehabilitation or another registered charity. In the event The Medical Disability Society was formed separate from the Society for Research. The Council agreed to these arrangements and agreed that 50% of the ordinary fund and 50% of the Trust fund should go to this new Society.

Rheumatology and General Medicine

Apart from the need for every rheumatologist to have a sound basic training in general medicine which was always agreed, the needs of the rheumatology consultant for a commitment to general medicine has been debated over the years. Differing views have been expressed and it has been agreed that the specialty covers a wide spectrum and that training should also be broad based. It has been agreed that the exact responsibilities of a consultant post will rest with individual districts and some districts might not wish to appoint a rheumatologist without a commitment to general medicine. In the

informal meetings between individuals took place at times during the following years but it was not until 1977 that further more official efforts were made to improve the liaison between the BARR and the Heberden Society. Meetings took place between the President and Secretary of the BARR (Dr AT Richardson and Dr D Zutshi) and the President and Secretary of the Heberden Society (Professor V Wright and Dr JD Goode); Dr PHN Wood was co-opted after the first few meetings. The first meeting of this group was unofficial but after this the group became an official working party. The time seemed ripe for such discussions as members of both societies were finding it increasingly difficult to attend the meetings of both societies which covered very similar grounds and the cost of travel in time and money was increasing. Furthermore it was shown that there was a marked overlap in membership (60% of the total UK membership of BARR were also members of the Heberden Society and 63% of the clinical UK membership of the Heberden Society were members of the BARR). After preliminary meetings it was felt that the views of members should be ascertained and the Presidents wrote to the members of their respective societies. Some 70% supported a merger between the two societies and a further 15% were keen on further joint meetings, only 5% were against any sort of combination. A number of members of BARR were concerned about the non-rheumatological rehabilitation commitment of the association until a medical rehabilitation society could be established. It was noted in this respect that a society for research in rehabilitation had come into being and had held one meeting. It was also noted that a working party of the SAC of the JHMT of the RCP was considering the setting up of a separate SAC in rehabilitation.

The working party observed that whilst the aims of the two societies were the same, the Heberden Society was a learned scientific society devoted to rheumatology and its membership included those who were not clinicians. On the other hand, BARR had developed from physical medicine and whilst many consultants practised rheumatology, its members were also concerned with rehabilitation of the physically disabled. The Association was also a representative body concerned with the professional interests of rheumatologists in the manner of a trade guild. They organised training programmes and were concerned with the recruitment, distribution and facilities of staff and were involved in teaching of other related subjects (ie EMG techniques, paediatrics, soft tissue lesions and sports injuries). These facts were collected into an interim report issued in June 1978 with the recommendations that:

(1) Serious considerations should be given to closer liaison between the two bodies;
(2) Regular combined meetings were a desirable feature;
(3) The BARR should issue an invitation to clinical members of the Heberden Society to attend the 1979 AGM for a general discussion on the issue;

(4) The Heberden Society extend an invitation to members of BARR to attend scientific discussions at the 1978 AGM;
(5) The working party should remain with the same membership to continue deliberations and review progress.

In addition, there should be a joint secretariat. The BARR AGM of April 1979 endorsed these recommendations and the Executive of the Heberden Society asked for a more far reaching document putting forward concrete proposals on closer co-operation between the two societies. The working party therefore continued its work and were joined by Dr JT Scott who was now President of the Heberden Society. Professor V Wright was now President of BARR. They drew up a draft constitution entitled 'Professional Associations Concerned with Rheumatology and Rehabilitation'. This visualised a federated arrangement with BARR continuing its professional, political and education role and adopting a 'trade guild' function with the Heberden Society continuing its scientific function and possibly other bodies such as the ARC and the Rehabilitation Society affiliated to the BARR.

In the event both the Council of BARR in February 1979 and the Heberden Executive rejected the proposals, but a simpler interim proposal put forward by Dr G Panayi was accepted. This suggested that:

(1) the two societies should have cross representation on each others councils or executive committees;
(2) joint annual meetings should be formally recognised;
(3) there should be a joint secretariat to be set up as soon as practicable;
(4) the more controversial aspects of federation should remain for discussion by the working party.

The membership of the working party changed from time to time over the next year and whilst the first two proposals were easy to fulfil *viz* cross-representation of members and joint annual meetings, the joint secretariat was more difficult because of lack of space particularly at the RCP. However, by October 1981 the two societies had established a joint secretariat at 41 Eagle Street, Holborn in premises purchased by the Arthritis and Rheumatism Council. By this time however the climate of opinion had changed and the working party now recommended that there should be a merger of the two societies–that the BARR and Heberden Society should be dissolved and they should be replaced by a single society, the name of which was to be established. The change in climate seems to have been due to the fact that rehabilitation was now accepted as a separate discipline and related to general (internal) medicine with a society capable of surviving in its own right and that it would not figure in the commitment of the new society.

The working party now concentrated entirely on the constitution of the new society. The constitution which was decided upon did not differ greatly from those the parent societies suggested: that there should be Full, Retired, Overseas and Honorary Members. Full

Members would be elected by the Council. The Society would be open to all scientific and professional workers in rheumatology and non-medical qualified scientists. Annual scientific meetings should be held every year normally in London. Additional scientific and educational meetings should be held as determined by the Council. An AGM should be held on the occasion of the Annual Scientific Meeting.

The Honorary Officers should be a President, a President-elect, an Immediate Past President, a Treasurer, a Secretary, an Assistant Secretary, a Deputy Secretary, Editor and Heberden Librarian. The President-elect would hold this office for 1 year after which the member would become President for 2 years and then for another year be Immediate Past President. The Treasurer would serve for 3 years.

The Assistant Secretary would hold office for 1 year and then would be the Secretary for 2 years after which the member would be the Deputy Secretary for a further year. The Council would consist of twelve elected members serving 3 years.

It was envisaged that there would be three standing sub-committees: (1) Clinical Affairs Committee (medical only), (2) Scientific Meetings Committee, and (3) Education Committee.

Junior staff would be represented on the Council and in Standing Committees. The name Heberden would be preserved in the Heberden Round, Heberden Oration and Heberden Library. The New Society would seek charitable status.

There was some discussion about the journals. The *Annals of the Rheumatic Diseases* had been the official journal of the Heberden Society—it was a specialised journal of the BMA whilst *Rheumatology and Rehabilitation* was owned by the BARR and published by Baillière Tydall & Cox Ltd, profits being shared between the publishers and the Association. It was agreed that there was a place for both journals and the working party recommended that members should receive both journals. In the event *Rheumatology and Rehabilitation* became the *British Journal of Rheumatology* and the official journal of the Society whilst the *Annals* had to be purchased separately from the BMA.

The proposed constitution was now presented to a joint meeting of the Heberden Executive and the BARR Council on 10 March 1982. There were only minor changes made and the working party was authorised to proceed with a time table for the merger of the two societies in the British Society for Rheumatology (BSR). The working party over this period had been Dr JT Scott (Chairman), Dr G Panayi, Dr BEW Mace, Dr Jean Colston, Dr Rodney Grahame, Dr NJ Sheehan, Dr ML Snaith, Dr Philip Wood, Mr MCG Andrews, Professor V Wright, Mrs J Seeds and Miss Carol Stevens (Executive Secretaries). Professor D Brewerton and Dr DHH Yates became members later with Miss R Broke-Evans and Mr J Nortin in attendance. The working party had further meetings and the Council of the BARR had further discussions and it was agreed that the draft constitution

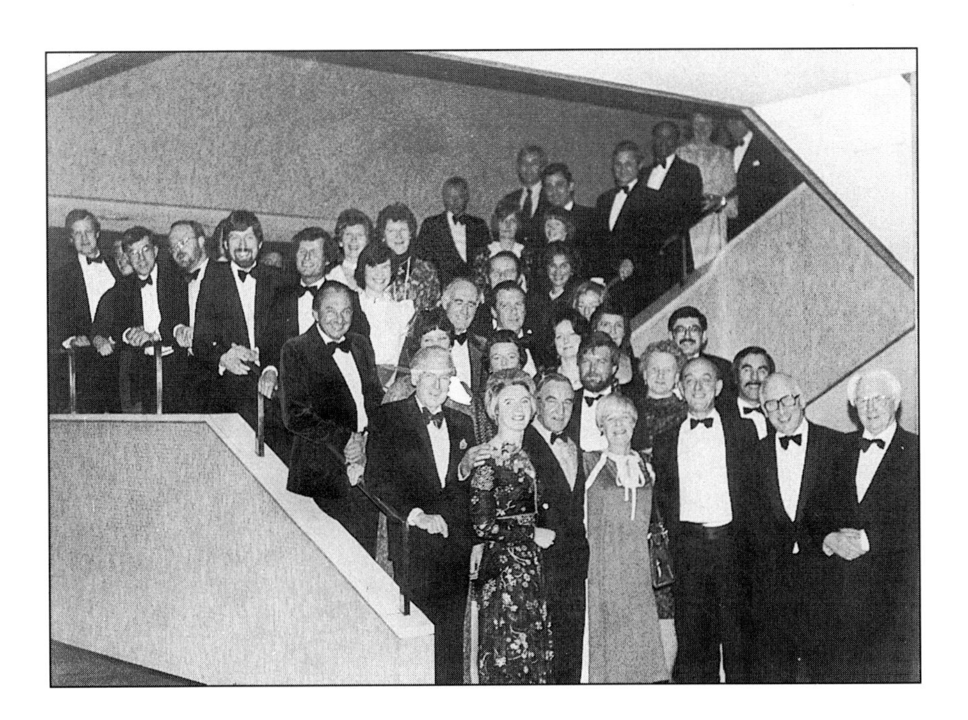

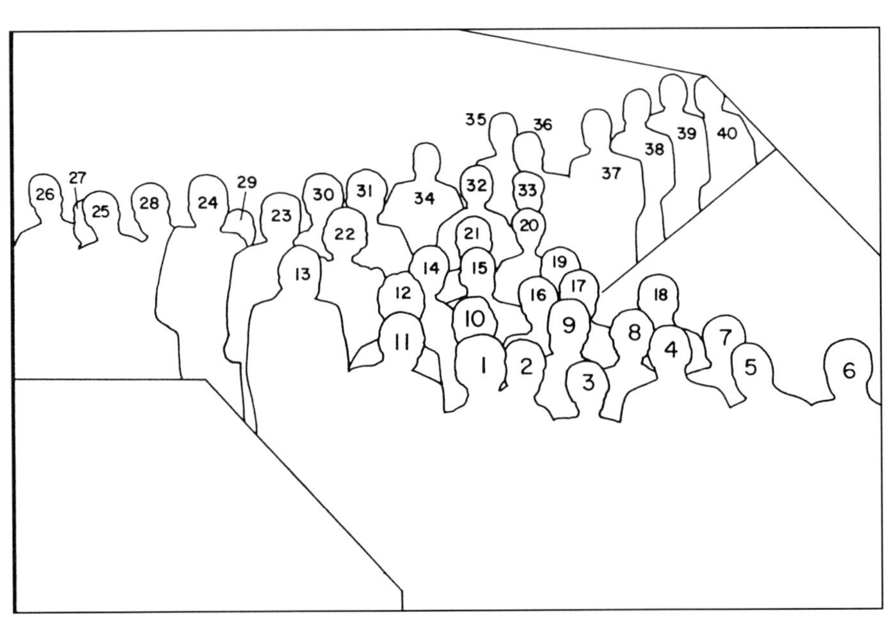

Retirement dinner for Dr AC Boyle, 15 April 1983 at the Royal College of Physicians

1 BW Mace; 2 DL Woolf; 3 D Hayley; 4 M Corbett; 5 AC Boyle; 6 Mrs Boyle; 7 CE Quin; 8 J Colston; 9 C Williams; 10 M Shipley; 11 S Jones; 12 unknown; 13 A Bamji; 14 C Dunn; 15 S Hodgson; 16 unknown; 17 W Williams; 18 I Williams; 19 L Marks; 20 J Evans; 21 P Woolf; 22 A Young; 23 E Kauffman; 24 J Winfield; 25 N Cox; 26 FW Webb; 27 J Halsey; 28 unknown; 29 R Barter; 30 J Spurr; 31 unknown; 32 D Rolfe; 33 M Seifert; 34 F Bruckner; 35 A Chamberlain; 36 A Ebring; 37 N Pandit; 38 H Kerr; 39 unknown

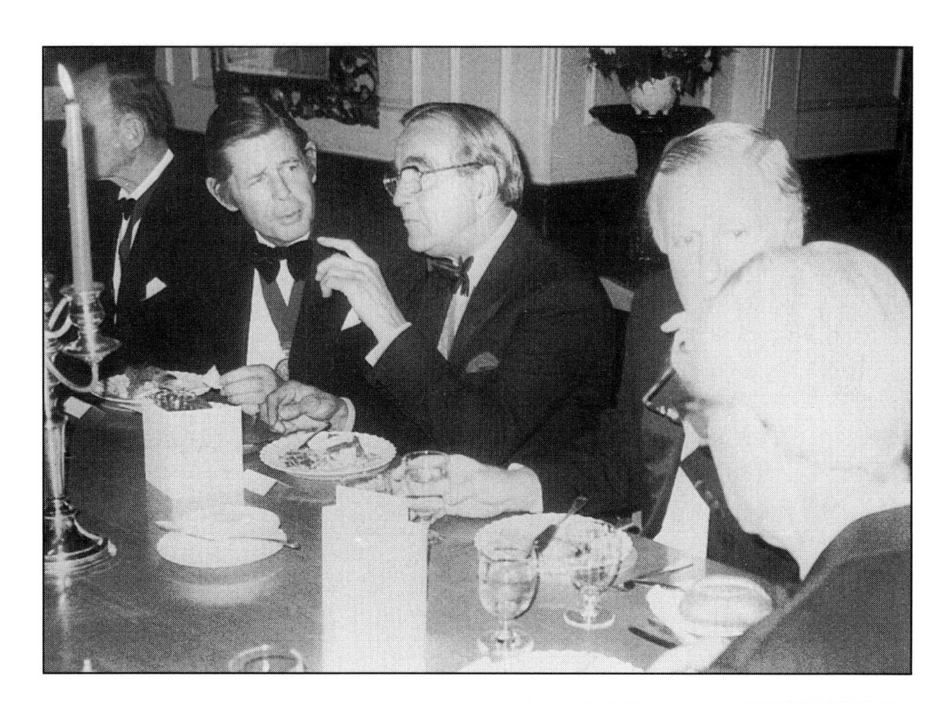

Presidents, DAH Yates, AC Boyle, AT Richardson

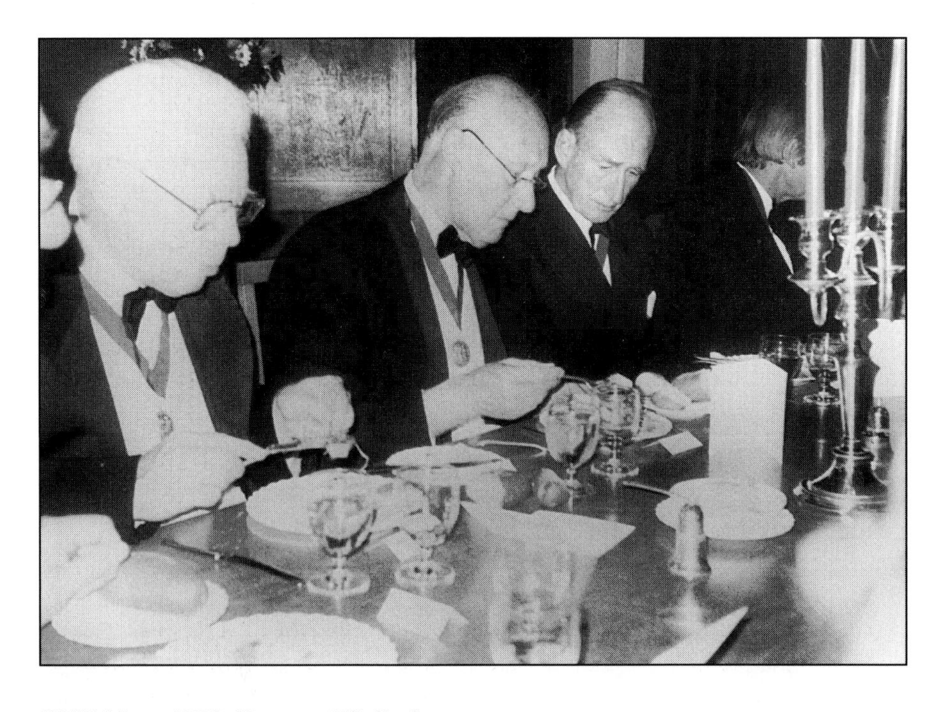

BEW Mace, DRL Newton, FS Cooksey

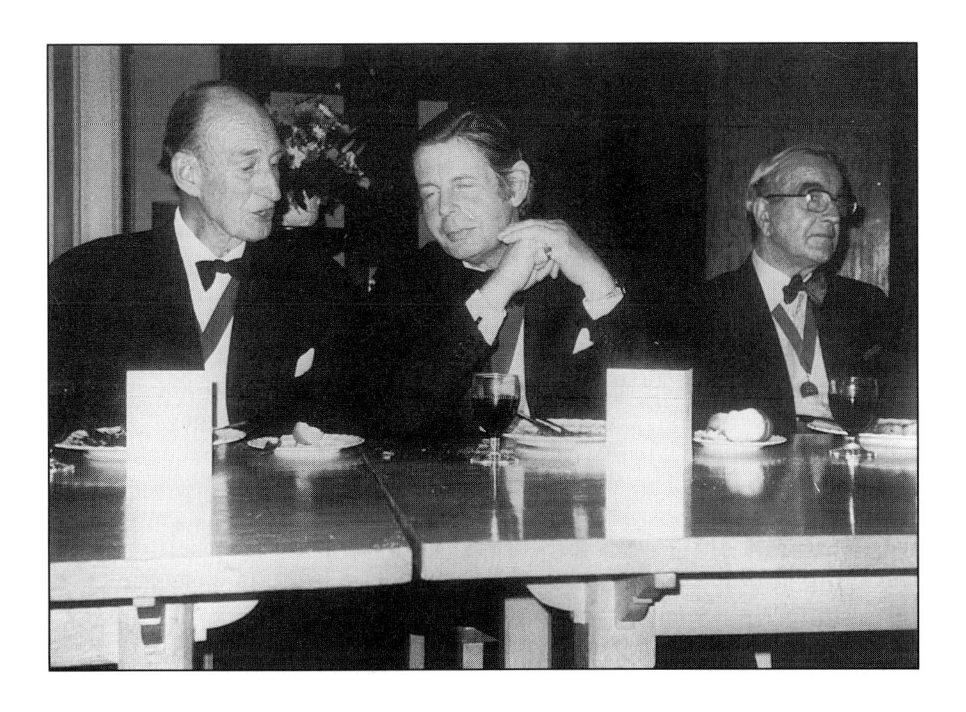

FS Cooksey, AH Yates, AC Boyle

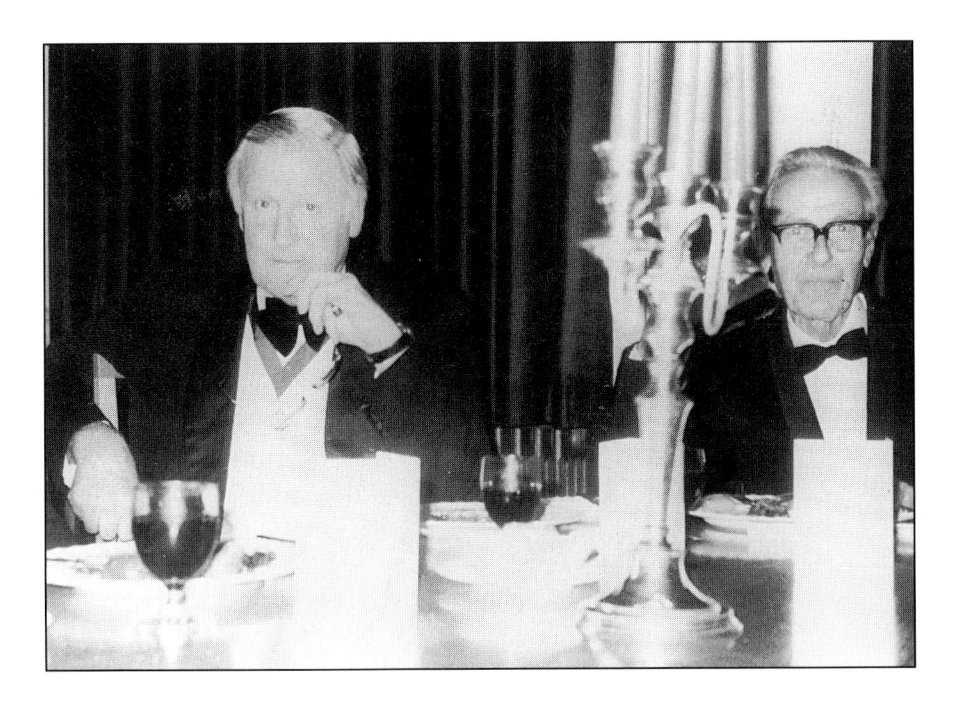

AT Richardson with GD Kersley

should be sent to all classes of membership and a postal ballot of Full and Associate Members concerning the acceptance of the constitution should be held synchronously with a ballot of members of the Heberden Society. It was also necessary to get the agreement of the Charity Commissioners on the establishment of the new society's funds and the 50/50 division of the BARR and the Research and Education Trust fund with the corresponding rehabilitation society. In May 1983 the result of the postal ballot was reported. For BARR 198 Members and Associate Members had voted in favour of dissolution, 35 voting against. For the Heberden Society 467 had voted in favour with 38 against. A further joint meeting between the BARR Council and the Heberden Executive took place in July 1983. It was decided that members and officers of the two bodies who still had remaining terms of office to run would form the governing body of the new society and in addition there would be five vacancies. A postal ballot for the President of the new society was arranged and Professor G Nuki was elected. In an editorial in the *British Journal of Rheumatology*, Dr R Grahame welcomed the new Society with the reasons for the amalgamation, and the hope that the society would give its wholehearted support to its members in the new society for rehabilitation. A dinner for past and present members of the Council of BARR was held at the invitation of Dr DAH Yates, the last president at St Thomas's Hospital, on 19th October 1983 and 35 members attended. The two societies fused as from 1st January 1984 as the British Society of Rheumatology.

Appendices

Physical Treatments in Use in the 1930s

Baths
Climatology—general principles—factors influencing health and disease
Diathermy and short-wave
Electrotherapy—galvanism and faradism
Heliotherapy
High frequency currents
Hydrology—use of water in treatment of disease
Light and heat
Massage—touching techniques
Massage and manipulations
Mineral waters—therapeutic use
Occupational therapy
Packs
Pool baths
Pyretotherapy
Radiant heat and infra-red
Remedial exercises
Ultra-violet light
Under water manipulation

Officers of the British Association of Physical Medicine and British Association of Rheumatology and Rehabilitation

	1943	1950	1952
President	Lord Horder	Lord Horder	Lord Horder
Vice President		Dr P Bauwens	Dr P Bauwens
Hon Treasurer	Dr MB Ray	Dr FS Cooksey	Dr WS Tegner
Hon Secretary	Dr P Bauwens	Dr WS Tegner	Dr AC Boyle
Hon Editor	Dr MB Ray (1947)	Dr HA Burt	Dr HA Burt

	1954	1955	1957
President	Lord Horder	Lord Horder	Dr P Bauwens
Vice President	Dr WS Tegner	Dr WS Tegner	Dr HA Burt
Hon Treasurer	Dr P Bauwens	Dr AC Boyle	Dr D Wilson
Hon Secretary	Dr AC Boyle	Dr GO Storey	Dr GO Storey
Hon Editor	Dr HA Burt	Dr HA Burt	Dr AC Boyle

	1959	1962	1965
President	Dr HA Burt	Dr WS Tegner	Dr FS Cooksey
Vice President Senior	Dr P Bauwens	Dr HA Burt	Dr WS Tegner
Vice President Junior	Dr WS Tegner	Dr FS Cooksey	Dr AC Boyle
Hon Treasurer	Dr J Shulman	Dr KN Lloyd	Dr DR Newton
Hon Secretary	Dr AT Richardson	Wing Comm CB Wynn Parry MBE	Dr A Brewerton
Hon Editor	Dr AC Boyle	Dr AC Boyle	Dr P Hume Kendall

	1966	1968	1970
President	Dr FS Cooksey	Dr RM Mason	Dr RM Mason
Immediate Past President	Dr WS Tegner	Dr FS Cooksey	
Vice President		Dr HA Burt	Dr HA Burt
Vice President Junior	Dr AC Boyle		
Hon Treasurer	Dr DR Newton	Group Captain CB Wynn Parry	Group Captain CB Wynn Parry
Hon Secretary	Dr DA Brewerton	Dr PJ Nichols	Dr APH Randle
Ass Hon Secretary	Dr PJR Nichols	Dr APH Randle	Dr DAH Yates
Hon Editor	Dr P Hume Kendall	Dr P Hume Kendall	Dr DL Woolf

	1972	1973	1974
President	Dr AC Boyle	Dr AC Boyle	Dr DRL Newton
Immediate Past President	Dr RM Mason	Dr RM Mason	Dr AC Boyle
Vice President	Dr PJR Nicholls Dr DRL Newton		
Hon Treasurer	Dr GO Storey	Dr GO Storey	Dr R Grahame
Hon Secretary	Dr DAH Yates	Dr R Grahame	Dr TA Matthew
Assis Hon Secretary	Dr R Grahame	Dr JA Matthews	Dr DW Zutshi
Immediate Past Secretary			Dr JA Matthews
Hon Editor	Dr DL Woolf	Dr DL Woolf	Dr DL Woolf

	1975	1977	1978
President	Dr DRL Newton	Dr A Richardson	Prof V Wright
Immediate Past President	Dr AC Boyle	Dr DRL Newton	Dr AT Richardson
Hon Treasurer	Dr R Grahame	Dr JA Cosh	Dr JA Cosh
Hon Secretary	Dr DW Zutshi	Dr DW Zutshi	Dr M Corbett
Assis Hon Secretary	Dr GM Cochrane	Dr M Corbett	Dr DW Zutshi
Hon Editor	Dr DL Woolf	Dr DL Woolf	Dr DL Woolf

	1979	1980	1982
President	Dr BEW Mace	Dr BEW Mace	Dr DAH Yates
Immediate Past President	Prof V Wright	Prof V Wright	Dr BEW Mace
Hon Treasurer	Dr JA Cosh	Dr AK Tyler	Dr AK Tyler
Hon Secretary	Dr AWT Eade	Dr AWT Eade	Dr JR Colston
Deputy Hon Secretary	Dr M Corbett	Dr JW Colston	Dr DI Haslock
Hon Editor	Dr DL Woolf	Dr DL Woolf	Dr R Grahame

Presidents of the British Association of Physical Medicine and British Association of Rheumatology and Rehabilitation

1945–1955	The Lord Horder
1956–1959	Dr P Bauwens
1959–1962	Dr H Burt
1962–1965	Dr WS Tegner
1965–1968	Dr FS Cooksey
1968–1971	Dr RM Mason
1971–1974	Dr AC Boyle
1974–1976	Dr DRL Newton
1976–1978	Dr AT Richardson
1978–1980	Professor V Wright
1980–1982	Dr BW Mace
1982–1983	Dr DAH Yates

Common Abbreviations

AGM	Annual General Meeting
ARC	Arthritis and Rheumatism Council
BAPM	British Association of Physical Medicine
BARR	British Association of Rheumatology and Rehabilitation
BMA	British Medical Association
BMJ	*British Medical Journal*
BSR	British Society for Rheumatology
CSP	Chartered Society of Physiotherapists
DHSS	Department of Health and Social Security
D Phys Med	Diploma of Physical Medicine
DRO	Disablement Resettlement Officer
ECT	Electroconvulsive Therapy
EMG	Electromyography
EMS	Emergency Medical Service
ERC	Empire Rheumatism Council
IRU	Industrial Rehabilitation Unit
ISMH	International Society of Medical Hydrology
NHS	National Health Service
RCP	Royal College of Surgeons
RSM	Royal Society of Medicine
SMHO	Senior Medical Health Officer

Acknowledgements
I am very grateful to my colleagues for all their help. Particularly to Dr JMH Moll and Dr DL Scott for reading the script and for their advice. Dr AC Boyle has been very helpful. Many others have given me access to their records: Dr GD Kersley, Dr R Grahame, Dr BW Mace, Dr DRL Newton, Dr AT Richardson, Professor PHN Woods and Dr D Zutshi. Photographs have been supplied by Dr J Colston, Mr M Corbett, Dr EBD Hamilton, Dr JD Perry, Dr S Rudge and Dr DL Woolf. Advice has been given by Dr EDR Campbell, Dr EN Glick, Mr P Styles, Dr MG Wright, Professor V Wright, Dr CB Wynn-Parry and Dr CG Barnes.

I am extremely grateful for the secretarial work provided by Ms Shinaz Somoni and Ms Gina Tempalski.

I am grateful to Wesley's Chapel, City Rd, London for their permission to publish the Wesley material and the help given by the Archive Department at the Royal London Hospital and the Archive Department of St Bartholomew's Hospital, London for permission to publish the frontispiece.

References

My main sources are the minutes of the Council and Sub-committees of the BAPM, later the BARR. I have also had access to the minutes of the Physical Medicine (later Rheumatology and Rehabilitation) Group of the BMA; the minutes of the Duchenne Society and the Howitt Society; the minutes of Standing Advisory Committees to the RCP of Physical Medicine, Rheumatology and Rehabilitation.

Introduction

Moll JMH. The Heberden Society. Cambridge: University Press, 1987.

Chapter 1

The Spas

Allbutt The Rt Hon Clifford. Preface. *Arch Med Hydrol*, 1925: **1**; 1.

Bain W, Edgecombe W. *Harrogate baths and climate.* London: Longman Green, 1905.

Buckley CW. Osteoarthritis and its relation to chronic rheumatism. *Proc RSM*, 1911: **4 part 1**; 23.

Buckley CW. Painful affections of the shoulder. *Proc RSM*, 1914: **7 part 1**; 59.

Edgecombe W. Treatment of wounded and invalid soldiers. *Arch Med Hydrol*, 1924: 1-2: 140.

Foster MG. *Baths and Mineral Waters of Britain and Europe.* Bristol: John Wright, 1933.

Fox RF. Outlines of medical hydrology. *Proc RSM*, 1910: **4**; 63.

Gordon W (Chair). Discussion on the treatment by physical methods of disabilities induced by war. *Proc RSM*, 1916–17: **10 part 1**; 1.

Gowers Sir W. Lumbago: its lessons and analogues. *Br Med J*, 1904: **1**; 117.

Hernaman-Johnson F. On the value of combined methods of diagnosis. *Proc RSM*, 1920–21: **14 part 1**; 23.

Horder The Lord. Rheumatism: a national problem. *Ann Rheum Dis*, 1952: **12**; 1.

Howitt FD. The evolution of physical medicine. *Proc RSM*, 1952: **45**; 458.

Kersley GD. *The Three Rs.* Bath: Ralph Allan Press, undated.

Llewellyn Jones. Arthritis deformans. *Proc RSM*, 1910: **3 part 1**; 85.

Llewellyn JL. A discussion on fibrositis. *Proc RSM*, 1913: **6 part 1**; 27.

Newton DRL. The complete rheumatologist. *Proc RSM*, 1973: **66**; 15.

Rolls R. *The Hospital of the Nation.* Bird Publications, 1988, pp 1, 128.

Section of Physical Medicine. Meeting report. *Proc RSM*, 1931: **25 part 1**; 321.

Tegner WS. A short history of the BAPM&R. *Rheum Phys Med*, 1972: **11**; 210.

Physical Therapy

Anon. *The Medical Directory 1931.*

Burt H. Editorial. *Ann Phys Med*, 1952: **1**; 2.

Copeman WSC. Historical notes on rheumatism. *Rheum Phys Med*, 1971: **11**; 145.

Graves C. *The Story of St Thomas' Hospital 1106–1947*. Faber & Faber, 1947, p 56.
Hume-Kendall P. Editorial. The origins of physical medicine. *Ann Phys Med*, 1965: **8**; 1.
Jewesbury ECO. *The Royal Northern Hospital.* HK Lewis, 1956.
Kersley GD. *The Three Rs.* Bath: Ralph Allen Press, undated.
McInnes EM. *St Thomas' Hospital.* London: George Allen Unwin, 1963, p 163.
Mennell JB. The tradition of physical medicine. *Ann Phys Med*, 1952: **1**; 151.
Morris EW. *A History of the London Hospital.* London: Edward Arnold, 1926, p 13.
Stanton-Wood Sir Robert. *Medical History of the Second World War.* London: HMSO, 1952, p 366.
Tegner W, Mason RM, Barnes CG. The London Hospital. The Department of Physical Medicine and Rheumatology. *Ann Phys Med*, 1970: **X**; 218.
Wesley John. *Primitive Physic or Easy and Natural Methods of Curing Most Diseases.* London: G Paramore, 1792, 24th ed.

Early Interest in Rheumatology

Anon. Clinics for rheumatism. *Br Med J*, 1927: **2**; 795.
Anon. Report. *Acta Rheum*, 1928: **1**; 1.
Anon. Leading article. Chronic rheumatism. *Br Med J*, 1932: **1**; 1086.
Anon. Report. *Acta Rheum*, 1938: **10**; 9.
Boyle AC. The Department of Rheumatology and Physical Medicine. *Rheum Phys Med*, 1972: **11**; 213.
British Red Cross Society. *The Campaign Against Rheumatism. Recommendation on the building equipments and staffing for a clinic for treatment of rheumatism.* London: BRCS, 1931.
Copeman WSC. Annual Report of the British Committee. *Rep Chr Rheum Dis*, 1935: **1**; 9.
Glover JA. Report to Minister of Health. Chronic arthritis with special reference to provision of treatment. *Rep Arch Med Hydrol*, 1922: **1–2**; 6, 44.
Glover JA. *Ministry of Health Reports on Public Health. The Incidence of Rheumatic Disease.* London: HMSO, 1924.
Glover JA. Report to Minister of Health. Chronic arthritis with special reference to provision of treatment. *Rep Arch Med Hydrol*, 1925–27: **3–5**; 76, 93, 121, 193, 233, 270.
Glover JA. Report to Minister of Health. Chronic arthritis with special reference to provision of treatment. *Rep Arch Med Hydrol*, 1928–29: **6–7**; 36, 98, 126, 165.
Glover JA. Report to Minister of Health. Chronic arthritis with special reference to provision of treatment. *Rep Arch Med Hydrol*, 1930–32: **8–9**; 280.
Kersley GD. *The Three Rs.* Bath: Ralph Allen Press, undated.
Moll JMH. *The Heberden Society.* Cambridge: University Press, 1987.
Newman Sir George. *Outline of the Practice of Preventive Medicine. Memorandum to the Minister of Health.* London: HMSO, 1926, p 94.
Willcox Sir W. Foreword. *Rheum Dis*, 1939: **1**; 1.
Wood PHN. Personal communication. 1988.

Electrodiagnosis

Adrian ED, Bronk DW. Impulses in motor nerve fibres. *J Phys*, 1929: **67**; 119.
Bauwens P. Electro-diagnosis and electrotherapy in peripheral nerve lesions. *Proc RSM*, 1941: **34**; 459.
Bauwens P, Richardson AT. *Recent Advances in Physical Medicine.* London: JA Churchill, 1950, p 6.
Buller AJ, Styles P. Technical factors affecting the accuracy of recording in EMG investigation. *Ann Phys Med*, 1952: **1**; 37.
Campbell EDR. Achievements of Duchenne. *Proc RSM*, 1973: **66**; 18.
Richardson AT. Clinical electromyography in the RAF. *Proc RSM*, 1949: **42**; 587.
Richter CP. The interpretation of the electromyogram from voluntary and reflex contractions. *Quart J Exp Physiol*, 1927: **18**; 55.
Styles P. Personal communications, 1989.
Wachholder. *Phluger's Arch*, 1923: 199; 595.
Weddell G, Feinstein B, Pottle RE. The electrical activity of voluntary muscle in man under normal and pathological conditions. *Brain*, 1944: **67**; 178.

Early Rehabilitation

Anon. *Report of the Joint War Committee of BRCS and Order of St John of Jerusalem in England (1914–1919).* London: HMSO, 1919.
Coulter JLS. *History of the Second World War. The Royal Navy.* London: HMSO, 1954, vol 1, p 370.
Jones Sir R, Girdlestone GR. The Cure of Crippled Children. *Br Med J* 1919: **2**; 457.
Kersley GD. *The Three Rs.* Bath: Ralph Allen Press, undated.
Millard JB. Voluntary organisations. *Rheum Rehab*, 1969: **10**; 440.
Nicholls TB. *Organisation, Strategy and Tactics of the Army Medical Service in War.* London: Baillière Tindall & Cox, 1937.
Patterson JWT. *Rehabilitation in the Army. Recent Advance in Physical Medicine.* London: JA Churchill, 1950, p 371.
Tegner WS. A short history of the BAPM&R. *Rheum Phys Med*, 1972: **11**; 210.
The British Red Cross Society. *Role of Hospitals for Treatment of Sick and Wounded Soldiers.* London: BRCS, Oct 1915.
Ward FG. Rehabilitation in the Navy. *Rheum Phys Med*, 1970: **10**; 428.
Watson F. *The Life of Sir Robert Jones.* London: Hodder & Stoughton, 1934.
Whittaker VB. Rehabilitation in the Army. *Ann Phys Med*, 1970: **10**; 428.
Woolf DL. Editorial. Rehabilitation. *Rheum Phys Med*, 1970: **10**; 385.
Wynn Parry CB. Some aspects of rehabilitation in the RAF. *Proc RSM*, 1954: **47**; 159.
Wynn Parry CB. Rehabilitation in the RAF. *Rheum Phys Med*, 1970: **10**; 428.

Physical Fitness

Newman Sir G. *An Outline of the Practice of Preventive Medicine (1919–1926). Memorandum to the Minister of Health.* London: HMSO, 1926.

Chapter 2
The Foundation and Structure of the British Association of Physical Medicine

Presidents and Presidential Badge

Anon. Obituary. Frank Howitt. *Ann Phys Med*, 1954: **2**; 73.
Anon. Obituary. Lord Horder. *Ann Phys Med*, 1955: **2**; 273.
Bauwens P. The Presidential Badge. *Ann Phys Med*, 1957: **4**; 1.
Mace BEW. Personal communication. 1989.
Wright V. Personal communication. 1989.

Annual General Meeting and Scientific Meeting

Joseph Sir Keith. Strategy for the development of the medical rehabilitation services. *Ann Rheum Rehab*, 1973: **12**; 105.

Chapter 3
Impact of the National Health Service

Editorial. Development of consultant services. *Br Med J*, 1952: **1**; 984, 1095.
Horder The Lord. *Fifty Years of Medicine*. London: Gerald Duckworth, 1955 (quoted in *Ann Phys Med*, 1955: **2**; 273).

Developments in Rheumatology

Anon. *Minutes of Executive Committee*. London: ERC, 1953, 1954.
Brain WR (chair). *Report of the Committee on Chronic Rheumatic Diseases*. London: RCP, 1957.
Hench PS, Kendall EC, Slocumb CG, Polley HF. *Proc Mayo Clinic*, 1949: **8**; 21.
Kersley GD. *The Three Rs*. Bath: Ralph Allen Press, undated.
Platt Sir Robert (chair). *Report of the Committee on Chronic Rheumatic Diseases*. London: RCP, 1961.

The Piercy Committee—Rehabilitation

Piercy Rt Hon Lord (chair). *Ministry of Labour and National Services Committee of Inquiry on Rehabilitation. Training and Resettlement of Disabled Persons*. London: HMSO, 1956.
Tomlinson G (chair). *Ministry of Labour and National Service Inter-departmental Committee on Rehabilitation and Resettlement of Disabled Persons*. London: HMSO, 1942.

Paramedical Services

Anon. Discussion. The Scientific Approach. *Ann Phys Med*, 1954–55: **2**; 5.
Anon. Editorial. Supplementary professions. *Br Med J*, 1960: **2**; 1375.
Hume-Kendall P. Editorial. Science in physical treatment. *Ann Phys Med*, 1966: **8**; 149.

The Porritt Committee—Medical Staffing Structure in the Hospital Services

Council of BMA. Report. *Br Med J*, 1963: **suppl 1**; 229.

Porritt Sir A (chair). *Joint Working Party in the Medical Staffing Structure in the Hospital Services. Review of the Medical Services in Great Britain.* London: Social Assay, 1962, p 127 (also recommended pp 502–518).
Tegner WS. Specialists in rehabilitation. *Br Med J*, 1962: **2**; 1320.
Tegner WS. Specialists in rehabilitation. *Lancet*, 1962: **ii**; 1052.

Chapter 4
The Journal

Burt H. Editorial. *Ann Phys Med*, 1952: **1**; 1.

Chapter 5
International Congress of Physical Medicine

Anon. Minutes of the Executive Council. *International Congress of Physical Medicine Press Reports.*

Chapter 6
Changing Demands on the Service

Physical Medicine and Rheumatology

Anon. Report on medical staffing in the NHS in England and Wales. *Lancet*, 1967: **ii**; 668.
Anon. Report on the medical staffing in the NHS in England and Wales. *Lancet*, 1968: **ii**; 448.
Scott JT. Career structure in rheumatology. *Ann Rheum Dis*, 1969: **28**; 662.
Zutshi D. Personal communication. 1990.

Tunbridge Committee

Anon. Editorial. Rehabilitation services. *Br Med J*, 1972: **2**; 727.
Tunbridge Sir Ronald. *Report of the Sub-committee of the Standing Advisory Committee.* London: HMSO, 1972.

Guide to Training

Anon. Report. *Ann Phys Med*, 1966: **8**; 273.

Chapter 8
Further Developments

Electrodiagnosis

Campbell EDR. Carpal tunnel syndrome. Report on method of measuring sensory and motor conduction in carpal tunnel syndrome. *Proc RSM*, 1962: **55**; 401.
Dawson GD, Scott JW. The recording of nerve action potentials through the skin in man. *J Neural Psych*, 1949: **12**; 259.
Gilliat RW, Sears TA. Sensory nerve action potentials with peripheral nerve lesions. *J Neurol Psych*, 1958: 21; 109.
Hordes R, Larrabee MG, German W. The human electromyogram in response to nerve stimulation and conduction velocity of motor axons. *Arch Neurol Psych*, 1948: **60**; 340.

The Remedial Professions

Anon. *Appendix District Therapist Managers, Job Description. HSC (79) 19*. London: HMSO, 1974.

Anon. *The Remedial Professions and Linked Therapies. HSC (15) 101.* London: Health Service Circular Interim Services, 1974.

Anon. *Relationship Between the Medical Profession and Remedial Professions. HSC (77) 33*. London: HMSO, 1977.

McMillan EL (chair). *A report of a Working Party set up by the Secretary of State for Social Services on the Remedial Professions*. London: HMSO, 1973.

Newton DRL. Letter. Medical and Remedial Relationships. *Physiotherapy*, 1976: **62**; 201.

The Royal Commission on the Health Service (1977)–The Merrison Committee

Merrison Sir AW (chair). *Report of the Royal Commission on the National Health Service*. London: HMSO, 1979.

Boyle AC (chair). *The Challenge of Arthritis and Rheumatism Report of the Working Party of BLAR*. London: BLARR, 1977.

Chapter 9
Related Societies

The Heberden Society

Barnes CG. Personal communication. 1989

Kersley GD. *The Three Rs*. Bath: Ralph Allen Press, undated.

Moll JMH. *The Heberden Society*. Cambridge: University Press, 1987.

Physical Medicine Section of the RSM

Anon. *Minutes of Council*. London: RSM.

British Association of Manipulative Medicine

Cyriax J. *Treatment by Manipulation and Massage*. London: Cassal, 1944. Vol 2.

Cyriax J. *Text Book of Orthopaedic Medicine. Soft Tissue Lesions*. London: Cassal, 1947, 1962. Vol 1.

Wright MG. Personal communication. 1990.

Back Pain Association and Back Pain Research Society

Dixon A St J. Progress and problems in back pain research. *Rheum Rehab*, 1973: **12**; 165.

Kellgren JH, Lawrence JS, Swann A. Rheumatic complaints in an urban population. *Ann Rheum Dis*, 1953: **12**; 5.

Kersley GD. *The Three Rs*. Bath: Ralph Allen Press, undated.